U.S. DEPARTMENT OF HOUSING AND URBAN DEVELOPMENT
THE SECRETARY
WASHINGTON, D.C. 20410-0001

Foreword

The Department of Housing and Urban Development has served as a clearinghouse of innovative ideas and solutions – both for families and the greater real estate industry – for dealing with the problem of lead-based paint in our living environment. Today, we are concentrating on broad, workable, and affordable solutions to the problem of lead contamination in housing and the prevention of childhood lead poisoning. We have had success – the number of children suffering from lead poisoning is down – but we must do more on the enforcement and education front. We believe we have a mandate to raise the awareness of American families about lead hazards in their homes, and how they can keep their children safe from lead poisoning.

As part of our drive, we are republishing *Maintaining a Lead Safe Home*, a clearly written "How-To" book that can give you critical information about lead risks in your home or apartment, and what you can do to safeguard your family from lead hazards. It covers in straightforward language everything a family, a landlord, or building owner needs to know about safely dealing with lead paint and other lead poisoning threats. It details steps an individual can take to minimize or eliminate the problem, and also what steps you should take if you decide to hire a professional to evaluate your situation or undertake actual lead hazard control work.

Lead poisoning is the number one environmental health hazard for children under the age of six. Most of those children are poisoned from deteriorated paint and contaminated dust and soil. Lead poisoning is preventable. This book will help keep America's children safe.

Sincerely,

Andrew Cuomo

HUD maintains a current list of licensed lead-based paint inspectors and abatement contractors, which you can receive by calling toll-free 1-888-LEADLIST, or on the internet at WWW.LEADLISTING.ORG.

You can also visit HUD's lead-based paint homepage at WWW.HUD.GOV/LEA for additional information.

Maintaining A Lead Safe Home

Dennis Livingston

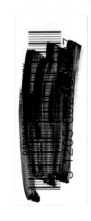

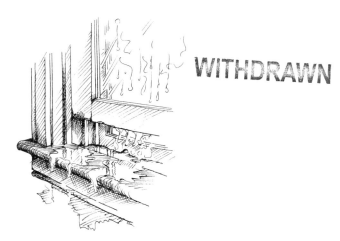

WITHDRAWN

For Information:

▼   ▼   ▼   ▼

DENNIS LIVINGSTON • COMMUNITY RESOURCES
28 EAST OSTEND STREET • BALTIMORE MD 21230
410-727-7837 • FAX 410-727-4242 • E-MAIL dlresource@aol.com

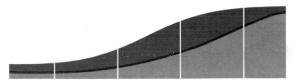

MAINTAINING A LEAD SAFE HOME
A Do-It-Yourself Manual for Home Owners and Property Managers
By Dennis Livingston

Published by:
Community Resources
28 East Ostend Street
Baltimore, MD 21230
Telephone: (410) 727-7837
Fax: (410) 727-4242
E-mail dlresource@aol.com

Reprinted by the U.S. Department of
Housing and Urban Development
Washington, D.C. 20410

Library of Congress Catalog Number: 97-94481

ISBN 0-9659833-0-7 (Paperbound)

ILLUSTRATIONS - Dennis Livingston
ART DIRECTOR - Carol Higgs, Gerson Higgs Design, Washington, D.C.
GRAPHIC DESIGN - Michael Fleckenstein, Spot Rock Inc., Baltimore., MD.
EDITING - Final editing by Lisa Platt. Initial editing by Susan McCallister,
 with funding support from the Alameda County Lead Poisoning
 Prevention Program, Oakland, CA.
PRINTING -

Printed in the United States of America

Credits & Acknowledgements

I wish to acknowledge the following people:

Charlie Doble, *whose pioneering work in lead paint introduced me to this field.*

Dr. Joan Luckhardt, *without whose persistence and patience this book would not exist.*

Steve Schwartzberg, Mark Delany, Anthony Von der Muhll *and* **Neil Gendel,** *who have put principles into practice.*

Dr. Mark Farfel *and* **David Jacobs,** *whose studies and publications have been critical in setting a standard in this field.*

Joe Lstiburek, *who has greatly enhanced my understanding of the house as a system.*

Dr. Warren Freedman *and* **Barbara Haley,** *who have been both mentors and critics of this book.*

I particularly wish to acknowledge the following individuals who have reviewed and commented on this book, and apologize for names I have left off:

Steven M. Schwartzberg *MPH,* **Laura Nicodemus** and **Douglas Henderson,** Alameda County Lead Poisoning Prevention Program • **Lynn M. Hermann** *M.A.,* Michigan Lead Poisoning Program Coordinator • **Kevin J. Sheehan,** Sheehan and Associates • **Ann Sheehan,** "The Courier" • **Joseph T. Ponessa** *Ph.D.,* Rutgers Cooperative Extension Service • **Anita Fong** • **Carena M. Thompson,** Liberty Family Learning Center • **Amy Frank** • **David Guthrie,** Center For Disease Control • **Karen Yu,** San Francisco Department of Health • **William Hamilton,** The Evergreen Group • **Alan Fairley** and **Margaret Olmsted** • **Richard Brooks,** Wisconsin Department of Health and Human Issues • **Robert Haug, Chrystene Wyluda** and **Diane Kinnane,** New Jersey Department of Community Affairs • **Lane Bailey,** Alameda County Housing and Community Development • **Bruce Lippy,** International Union of Operating Engineers • **Joe Schirmer,** Wisconsin Division of Health • **Dana Bress** and **Peter Ashley,** U.S. Department of Urban Development • **Don Ryan,** The Alliance to End Childhood Lead Poisoning (who read the manuscript while on his Florida vacation, no less) • **Richard Neuman** • **Caroline Mitchell,** Consumer Action.

Maintaining a Lead Safe Home

Contents

Contents

Introduction

This book's purpose is to equip parents, property owners, workers, and community activists with information they need to help solve the lead poisoning problem— affordably and safely for workers and the environment. Although the book's focus is on technical solutions, the author believes the major barrier to implementing effective, affordable solutions is political. There is a tendency for people who have entered a new field, early in its development, to monopolize knowledge and resources. There is also a tendency for agencies that are the recipients of lead program money to spend most of it on reaction and the rest on administrative expenses. Every carpenter, mother, do-it-yourselfer, painter, contractor, father, real estate agent, doctor, and daycare provider urgently needs to understand both the problem and the solution or we will not stop the poisoning.

An environmental problem that robs one out of 23 U.S. children of their potential is a national disaster. We have vastly greater resources and knowledge than is being applied. In fact, very little poisoning prevention (as opposed to reacting to poisoned children) is being implemented nationally. The author believes three policy shifts are necessary to solve this problem.

1. **Shifting away from reacting to poisoned children with expensive and often unnecessary full abatements, while shifting toward preventing poisoning.** We need to develop prevention programs that locate and solve housing maintenance problems before they damage the house or poison children. A woman's pregnancy or a change in occupancy are excellent prevention opportunities.

2. **Ending the chaotic practice of the "environmental problem of the decade."** Each time communities build the capacity to solve one environmental problem, policy makers declare a more urgent problem— energy conservation to asbestos to radon to lead to respiratory disease to ... ?

Introduction

Residential environmental problems are inextricably related. Moisture in a wall cavity is a source for lead poisoning, respiratory disease, higher energy bills and structural damage. A cost-effective, responsible program would provide holistic solutions to interrelated problems.

3. **Ending the delivery of services to community homes by large centralized bureaucracies.** Communities become reliant on government services and local services are put out of business.

The option is to use federal funds to build the capacity of community-based contractors, maintenance workers and painters to solve their own environmental problems as well as market their expertise to other communities. This creates jobs, develops a sustainable entrepreneurial infrastructure, and reverses the communities' dollar drain—all for a far lower cost.

It is the author's hope that this book can be a tool in the hands of parents, community activists, and small property owners who wish to stop the poisoning of children, while also protecting workers and the environment and maintaining affordable housing.

Dennis Livingston
Baltimore, 1997

How to Use This Book

This is a How-to-Do-It Book on Preventing Lead Poisoning

This book is designed to give you critical information about lead hazard risks and what you can do about them. Some of the most detailed topics, such as how to take lead dust samples, are in appendices at the back of the book. This has been done so you can get an overview of the subject before reading about details.

The book is not designed to substitute for training or required state certification. But for people living in or doing work on old houses, this is critical information.

The color **RED** is used throughout the book to highlight important information such as a situation or action that may create a risk. In illustrations, **RED** draws attention to potential lead hazards.

🚫 This international symbol means that a method or action is prohibited.

Ⓐ This symbol is used when more detail on this subject is found in an appendix. The letter tells you which appendix.

① This symbol refers to footnotes at the end of the book.

Maintaining Family Health

Chapter 1

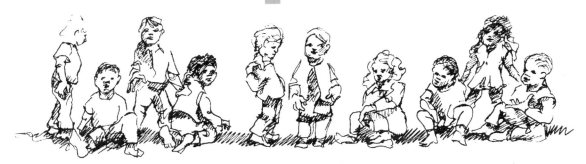

Nationally 1 out of 23 children has lead poisoning. According to the Center for Disease Control, 1 out of 6 low-income children, living in housing built before 1946, has lead poisoning. The damage to a poisoned child may be permanent. Poisoning can be prevented. **Most poisonings occur from exposure to paint that is failing due to poor maintenance!**

Maintain paint surfaces.

Dust test all old houses.

Keep areas where children play, sleep and eat particularly clean.

Have children tested.

Children tend to ingest more lead than adults, particularly young children crawling around on the floor putting things in their mouths. A small amount of lead also does more damage to children than to adults, as children's bodies are still developing.

A lead-poisoned child usually seems healthy. Most of these children are poisoned because they eat lead dust that has gotten on their hands, toys, food, pacifier, etc. **Damage is usually done before symptoms show.**

Sometimes children show signs of poisoning by:
- Changes in behavior • Physical problems
- Short attention span • Headaches
- Irritability/drowsiness • Stomach cramps
- Loss of appetite • Joint pains • Sleep disorders

If children are very sick they may also show these signs:
- Weakness/clumsiness • Frequent vomiting
- Loss of balance • Loss of skills • Convulsion

Children, six months to six years old, who may be exposed to a lead danger should be tested for elevated blood lead levels. **This is the only way to know if a child is poisoned.**

Lead paint that is intact and several layers down is <u>not a health risk</u> if it is maintained.

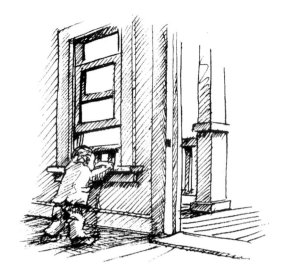

A child may be at risk of exposure if:

✔ The child spends time in a building built before 1978. This could be their home, daycare center, school, or baby sitter's.

✔ Renovation has been done to the house just before or during the time the child lived in the house.

✔ The child's house is near heavy industry or traffic where lead has contaminated the ground.

✔ A family member works with lead, like home restoration.

✔ The child ingests lead from lead-containing pottery or from folk medicines.

✔ A brother or sister's elevated blood lead levels may indicate a risk.

✔ The child plays in lead-contaminated soil.

✔ The child eats from lead-glazed dishes or chews on a lead-painted crib or toy.

✔ Water in the child's house is contaminated.

Test Children for Poisoning

A blood test tells you what a child's recent exposure to lead has been. Lead in blood is measured in micrograms of lead per deciliter of blood (µg/dL). A microgram is a millionth of a gram. A deciliter is about 3 ounces.

0	5	10	15	20	25	30	35	40	50	60	70

low risk   **moderate risk**   **high risk**   **urgent risk**

A level above 10 is of concern.
- Do a medical evaluation, including a test for iron deficiency.
- Recheck the child's blood level in a few months.
- Test the house for lead dust **A** or other lead risks.
- Address flaking and chipping paint, then clean up house and keep it clean. **B**

With a level above 15, do all of the above, plus:
- Begin medical management and more frequent testing.
- Remove child from lead hazard.

For a level above 20:
- Get a full medical evaluation for the child.
- Contact your local health department.
- Find and address the source of poisoning.

At higher levels of poisoning the child must be **immediately removed from hazard.** Medical treatment may be necessary.

What Poisons a Child?

The major cause of childhood lead poisoning is the child's normal hand-to-mouth activity like thumb sucking.

The major source of lead dust is painted surfaces that are flaking or chipping due to poor maintenance or renovation disturbance, and friction or impact surfaces, such as doors and windows.

Other major causes of poisoning are:
- Lead in soil, particularly bare soil, usually from exterior paint.
- Lead in drinking water.

Unless the causes of the paint failure are repaired and the failing paint is repaired and re-painted or sealed, a family cannot prevent poisoning.

Ways to Protect Children

There are measures that can be taken to help protect children before and after work is done:

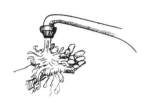

- Keep all painted surfaces intact.

- Keep children's hands clean. This is particularly important, especially before meals.

- Keep children's toys, particularly cloth toys, clothing, pacifiers, bottles and anything they might put in their mouths, clean.

- Keep children away from flaking paint and be sure it is not tracked through the house.

- Keep child away from any renovation work in your house or a neighboring house.

- Damp-clean areas where children spend time, particularly floors. This is of course difficult on a carpet. A regular vacuum cleaner may be used. If possible, borrow or rent a HEPA vac, it is a specialized vacuum cleaner that catches even the finest dust.①

- Make sure children eat a healthy diet. Although this is sometimes difficult, it is very important.

- Only cook and drink water from the cold water tap. Run for a couple of minutes before using.

- Try to keep children out of bare soil unless you have tested it and know it is safe.

- Have people take off shoes at the house entrance. At least have a door mat that people use. The mat should be cleaned frequently.

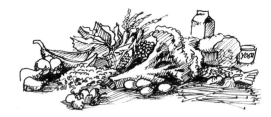

Diet

Eating food high in calcium and low in fat helps to keep a child from absorbing lead.

Some foods high in calcium are milk and foods made from milk (skim milk is best for children over two) and dark green vegetables like spinach and kale, etc.

Eating foods rich in iron is also important:
- dark greens (collards, broccoli)
- fish such as sardines and tuna
- bean and soy products like tofu
- eggs
- whole grains (rice, whole wheat bread, etc.)
- dried fruits (raisins, dates, prunes)
- lean meats and chicken (not deep-fried)

Avoid fatty foods such as:
- potato chips and other greasy snacks
- any deep-fried foods like french fries, batter-fried chicken, donuts, pastries, etc. (Save fast foods and sweets for special occasions.)

Have children eat at least three meals a day, particularly:
- fruits • whole grains • vegetables
- low-fat dairy products • beans • protein

This diet will also have many other health benefits.

> **A proper diet helps protect a child from lead poisoning.**

Adult Risk

Lead may also cause permanent damage to adults. Some major sources of risk to adults are:
- Working in a manufacturing industry that uses lead, such as a radiator repair or brass product industry.
- Renovating an old house. Demolition, sanding, burning or stripping paint are particularly dangerous.
- Working in the construction industry doing demolition or using lead in plumbing.
- Using lead in hobbies such as lead glass or casting bullets.
- Living in houses with extreme flaking and peeling paint.
- Eating food from containers soldered or glazed with lead or drinking liquids from lead crystal.

Workers exposed to lead or any other toxic substance who do not change out of their work clothes and clean themselves, may also expose their families.

The dust test reproduced below was from the car of a poisoned child's father. He drove co-workers home after working in a brass factory. Note: dust tends to cling to the stickiest place in a car.

TABLE 11
Results of Inspection for lead hazards: October, 1992 - Wisconsin.
Environmental Sampling

Sample Number	Area Sampled	Sample Results	Safe Levels
WS#1	Baby car seat	2,230 µg/ft²	< 200 µg/ft²
WS#2	Passenger car seat	67 µg/ft²	< 200 µg/ft²
WS#3	Driver car seat	228 µg/ft²	< 200 µg/ft²
WS#4	Car Driver floorboard	92 µg/ft²	< 200 µg/ft²
WS#5	Right work shoe	2,080 µg/ft²	< 200 µg/ft²
WS#6	Left work shoe	3,980 µg/ft²	< 200 µg/ft²
WS#7	Old work tennis shoe	890 µg/ft²	< 200 µg/ft²

It is not clear how low lead levels affect adults, but blood levels of 10 to 15 µg/dL can affect the fetus of a pregnant woman.

Adverse effects in adults at higher levels include:

- Abdominal discomfort
- Anemia
- Colic
- Constipation
- Excessive tiredness
- Fine tremors
- Headache
- High blood pressure
- Irritability or anxiety
- Loss of appetite
- Muscle and joint pain
- Pallor
- Pigmentation on the gums ("lead line")
- Sexual impotence
- Weakness
- Inability to keep hand and arm fully extended

Smoking, eating and drinking on a job that exposes workers to lead are particularly dangerous.

One way workers can find out if they are being exposed to lead dust on a job is to take a dust sample **A** from their work site and send it to a lab.

Survey the House

Chapter 2

> ✔ **The mere presence of lead paint does not mean there is a hazard.**

Test children's environment to find and eliminate risks of poisoning before children are exposed. This is a prevention strategy. The older the house, the more likely it is to be painted with lead paint.

Probability of a House Containing Lead

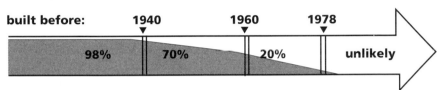

built before:	1940 ▼	1960 ▼	1978 ▼	
98%	70%	20%	unlikely	

Houses built before 1950 also had a higher percentage of lead in the paint.

The presence of lead paint that is stable, intact, undisturbed (particularly if it is covered by several layers of lead-free paint) is not, if maintained, a hazard.

To be able to test for and solve a lead problem, it is important to know the causes of the paint failure producing lead dust. This chapter will help you understand the various causes.

Doing a Visual Examination

To help determine if there is a lead risk you should visually examine your house, particularly porches, around windows and doors, exterior trim, and children's rooms.

Look for:
✔ flaking and peeling paint
✔ chipped paint
✔ places where paint is rubbed off
✔ weather-damaged paint

Taking Samples

To find out if there is a hazard of lead poisoning you can send a dust sample to a lab. The lab report will tell you how much lead is in the dust. Appendix **A** contains details of how to do this.

If an area is flaking, chipping, etc. or you are going to tear out a painted surface, do a chip test **A** to determine if paint is lead paint. You can also do a chemical test (also called a spot test kit), but they are not as accurate.

The most likely place for lead paint is exterior trim and siding. Inside the house, trim, particularly in the bathroom and kitchen, is most likely to be painted with lead paint. Those are also the two rooms most likely to have lead-painted walls. Other walls are least likely to contain lead.

Occupant Survey

Before we survey the house, there is some information you need about the home's history and its occupants:

Has there been any renovation or paint sanding, burning or scraping in the last few years?

If so, high dust levels may exist in the cracks of floorboards, carpets, and tops of cabinets. Collect dust wipes of surfaces that are not cleaned often. **A**

If there has been extensive exterior renovation or painting, take soil samples **A**, particularly if there is exposed soil on which a child plays.

Will improvements be made in the next few years? (for example, replacing windows or removing a wall)

If so, this work should be included as part of the work plan to reduce lead hazards.

Do adults have jobs with the possibility of lead exposure?

Wearing clothes home that contain lead dust can spread lead dust in the house or car.

Survey the House

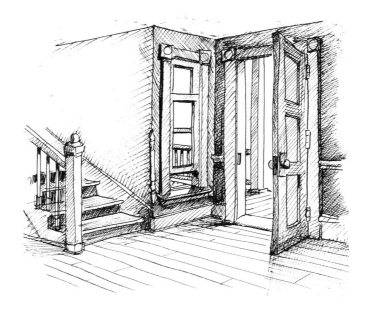

Do adults have hobbies, such as lead glass, casting lead or stripping furniture, that involve lead?

Where else does the child spend time, such as a daycare center, back yard, sand box, or another house the child visits often?

This is particularly important to know if your child has been exposed to lead and it appears your house is not the source, or the only source.

What are the ages and current blood lead levels of other children in the house?

If a child's blood lead level is near 10 µg/dL or higher, a "clean and stabilize" treatment may be prudent. This is described in Chapter 3 and Appendix **B**. Children must be out of the house during this treatment.

Hiring a professional

Instead of doing a survey yourself, you can hire a risk assessor for a more comprehensive investigation. See Chapter 4 for details.

Paint Failure

Again, the major cause of childhood lead poisoning is paint that is failing. Lead paint is usually several layers down. If not exposed, it does not create a danger.

To maintain safe, intact paint and to repair damaged paint, it is critical to understand the causes of paint failure:

- Moisture from inside and outside the house is the major cause of paint failure. It may also cause mold and mildew, which may cause respiratory disease.
- Friction and impact are the next most common causes.
- Other causes are poor surface preparation and, in relatively rare cases, children chewing on painted surfaces.

An old wall is made out of plaster on strips of wood called lath, nailed to wood studs.

The top layer of peeling paint is usually caused by incorrect surface preparation. The top layer peeling seldom exposes lead paint.

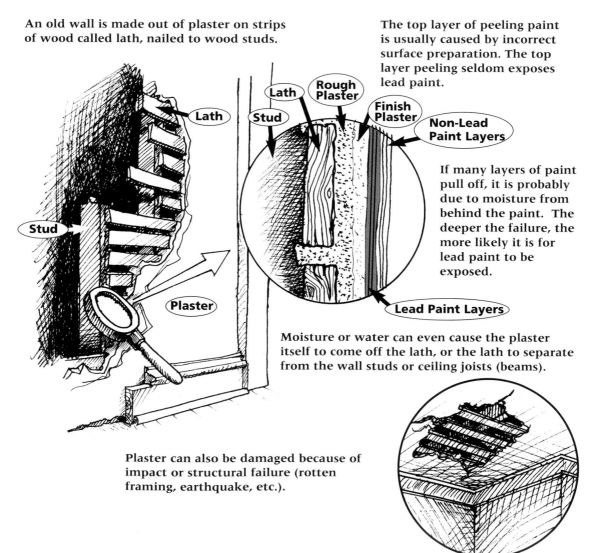

If many layers of paint pull off, it is probably due to moisture from behind the paint. The deeper the failure, the more likely it is for lead paint to be exposed.

Moisture or water can even cause the plaster itself to come off the lath, or the lath to separate from the wall studs or ceiling joists (beams).

Plaster can also be damaged because of impact or structural failure (rotten framing, earthquake, etc.).

Sources of Water and Moisture

In order to stop damage from water and moisture, you must locate their sources and develop a plan to solve the problem.

Gutters and downspouts that are clogged, leaking, or detached can cause wall damage. Check them by spraying roof with garden hose.

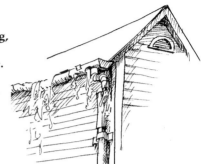

Roof Leaks - Water stains on a ceiling may indicate a roof leak. If accessible, check attic and roof.

Bathroom Problems - Be sure pipes or the seal around toilets doesn't leak.

Damaged Flashing - Flashing is the metal used to seal the space where a roof meets a wall or another roof, or the space around a vent, chimney or skylight. Keeping flashing in good shape is critical to keeping moisture out.

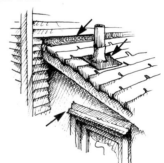

Kitchen - steam and moisture from cooking and cleaning can lead to paint failure.

Solution - vent to outside or open window when necessary.

Crawl Space - A wet crawl space can send moisture into house, which can cause paint failure and the growth of mold and mildew.

Solution - Keep dry, put plastic vapor barrier on dirt, insulate perimeter walls. In western and southern states install screened louvered vents for cross venting.

Basements - The moisture from dryers not vented to the outside can cause mold and mildew buildup and paint failure.

Solution - vent dryer to outside.

A downspout that dumps rain water at the foundation can create moisture problems in the basement. This is particularly true if the ground doesn't slope away from the house or the earth near the house is soft backfilled earth.

Solution - extend downspout, grade away from house and add splash block.

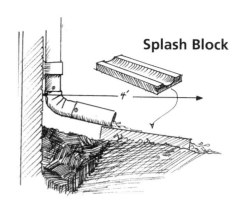

Splash Block

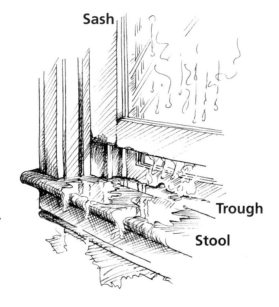

Sash

Trough

Stool

Water coming through the window can damage the stool (inside sill) and damage the wall and ceiling below.

Moisture can build up between the window and storm window. Water can be trapped by the storm window frame and collect in the trough. This can rot out the sill and damage the plaster under the window.

Solution - Drill two 1/4" holes in the bottom of the storm window frame, flush with the sill to let the water out.

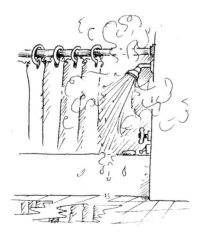

Showers create steam that, if not vented to the outside, can damage the ceiling and walls.

Solution - Install a vent fan or open a window.

Water splashed on a poorly sealed floor or leaking around tub because of poor caulking can damage the walls and ceiling below.

Before repairing damaged paint, it is <u>critical</u> to deal with the sources of moisture and water that are damaging the walls, ceilings, windows and trim. Preventing moisture damage will also prevent mold and mildew build-up.

See page 48 for a discussion of exterior paint.

Friction and Impact

When anything bangs into lead-painted wood or painted surfaces rub together, the top layers of non-lead paint are worn through or chipped away and lead dust or chips are created.

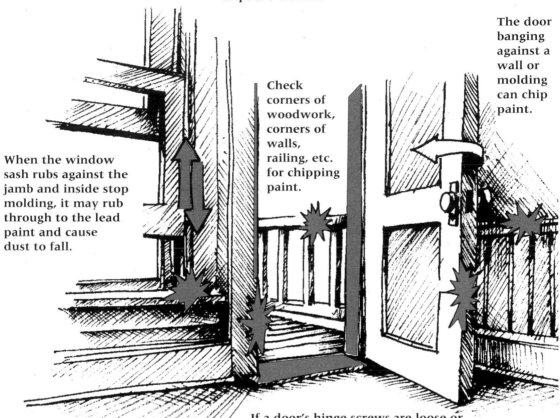

The door banging against a wall or molding can chip paint.

Check corners of woodwork, corners of walls, railing, etc. for chipping paint.

When the window sash rubs against the jamb and inside stop molding, it may rub through to the lead paint and cause dust to fall.

If a door's hinge screws are loose or the door rubs against the jamb (frame) or threshold, it can cause lead dust.

If the floor is painted with lead paint, the movement of toys and furniture and even people walking can cause lead dust. Sample any painted floor to see if it contains lead. A

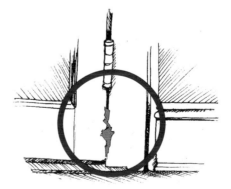

If a door makes contact with a door jamb on the hinge side when closed, it crushes the paint and produces lead dust.

Other Sources

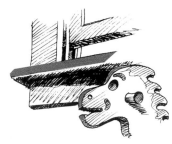

Chewable Surfaces

It is particularly important to inspect and possibly test easily chewable surfaces such as older painted wood. Children are most likely to put their mouths on round, protruding surfaces that are horizontal and at mouth height: window stools (inside sills), porch railings, painted toys, furniture (like a crib), or the nose of stair treads if they are lead painted. Testing is particularly important if the house is old (pre-1950) and these surfaces are flaking, chipping, or there are signs of children's tooth marks. You can test the paint with a chip or chemical test or hire a professional with an XRF machine.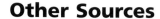

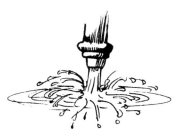

Water

The water in your house may contain elevated levels of lead. Water can pick up lead from either pipes or plumbing fixtures.

You should use water from the cold water tap—after letting it run for a while—for drinking, cooking or mixing formula. (It is particularly important to test water being used for formula.) Ask your municipal water department or bottled-water supplier if they have test results for lead in the water.

You can also test the water to see if it is safe. **A**
If there are dangerous levels of lead in your water:
- Buy a water filter that removes lead, or
- Use bottled water.

Renovation

If you have recently renovated a portion of your house (or you are currently doing so), you may have a lead hazard. Tearing out painted surfaces in old houses or removing paint will probably create high levels of lead dust. Sanding is particularly dangerous. If this kind of work has been done recently or is being done, remove children from the house, do dust tests **A**, and if the levels are high, seal and clean house. **B** You can do this work in a house where there is a child, if the work space is totally isolated. **C**

Survey the House

Never!

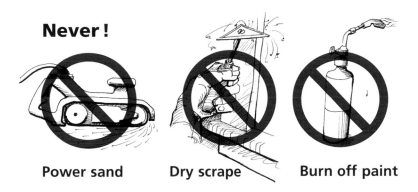

Power sand   Dry scrape   Burn off paint

Using chemical strippers in your home is also dangerous and should be avoided. Never use strippers containing **methylene chloride**. The use of heat guns is allowed if their temperature is kept below 1,100° Farenheit, but they are not effective at low temperatures and dangerous at high temperatures — their use is therefore discouraged.

Lead in Soil

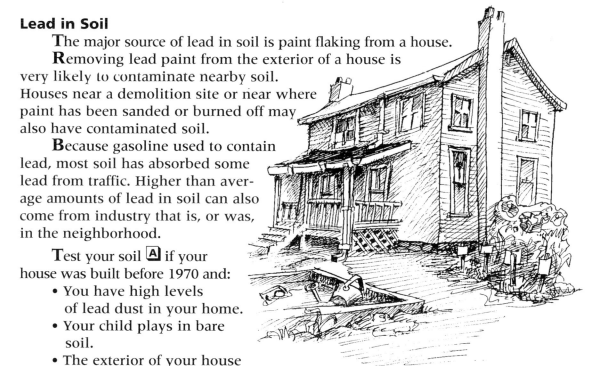

The major source of lead in soil is paint flaking from a house.

Removing lead paint from the exterior of a house is very likely to contaminate nearby soil. Houses near a demolition site or near where paint has been sanded or burned off may also have contaminated soil.

Because gasoline used to contain lead, most soil has absorbed some lead from traffic. Higher than average amounts of lead in soil can also come from industry that is, or was, in the neighborhood.

Test your soil **A** if your house was built before 1970 and:

- You have high levels of lead dust in your home.
- Your child plays in bare soil.
- The exterior of your house has been renovated or painted recently.
- You live near a factory, where a house has had the paint removed, or where a house has been demolished.
- You grow vegetables near an old house or near an industrial area.

To see if there may be lead-containing soil tracked into the house, take a dust sample at the entrance door. **A**

Survey the House

Bringing Home Lead Dust

If someone in the house works where lead is used, like a battery factory, or where lead dust is created, such as painting old homes or doing demolition, he or she may be bringing home lead dust. You can do a dust test on work shoes to see if there is a danger.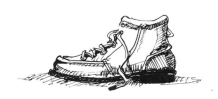

The hazard can be reduced if the worker wears protective clothing at work, changes clothes and washes hands before coming home, and showers when she or he get home or, if possible, before coming home.

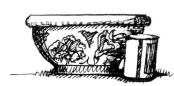

Containers

Containers may be tested with commercially available test kits.

- Glazed bowls with bright-colored glazes, particularly from outside the U.S., often contain dangerous amounts of lead.

- Crystal glassware may also contain lead. Never store wine in suspected lead crystal.

- Tin cans from outside the U.S., particularly those with wide grey seams, may have a high lead content. Never store food in open cans. Acidic food such as tomatoes, fruit juices, and vinegar draws out lead more easily than other foods.

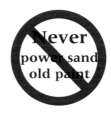

Hobbies

Some common hobbies can create an exposure to lead:

- casting lead into sinkers, bullets, etc.

- using leading in stained glass

- stripping and refinishing furniture (stripped furniture still contains lead)

If you do such hobbies at home, immediately test dust in your work area for lead. **A**
If levels are high:

- Test dust in the rest of the house.

- Keep children out of the work area.

- Do not eat, drink or smoke in the work area.
- Contain the work area. **C**

- Change clothes, particularly shoes, when leaving the work area (or remove protective clothing).

- Wash up every time you leave the work area.

- Keep the work area as clean as possible.

- Continue to monitor dust in and around the work area.

Notes

Stabilize, Clean and Maintain

Chapter 3

All work that breaks lead paint surfaces (painting, rehab, etc.) is lead work, no matter what it is called, and can be dangerous.

If you find a lead hazard in your home there is a great deal you can do yourself to solve the problem. This is a new field and there are few "professionals" available. Many of those who present themselves as experts have little experience, so it is good if you can understand your options.

The steps on any job are:
1. Identify the lead hazard.
2. Find the cause of damage and correct it.
3. Develop a plan to control the hazard.
4. Do the work safely and in a controlled space.
5. Clean up and take dust samples to be sure clean-up worked. Sampling may not be necessry where minuscule amounts of dust are created.
6. Monitor and maintain the property.

Work Options

Lead-poisoning prevention work has a wide range. Some measures, like cleaning, are simple. Others are more complex.

| Clean and Stabilize | Paint stabilization and hazard control | Hazard control as part of home improvement | Paint removal as part of "gut rehab" |

FROM: / **TO:**

Least expensive ▶ Most expensive
Least dangerous ▶ Most dangerous
Least skill required ▶ Most skill required
Shortest "life" ▶ Most permanent solution
Most need to monitor ▶ Least need to monitor

- Occupants and property owners can do some "clean and stabilize" work themselves.
- Additional work may be done by occupants and maintenance workers with skill in carpentry, cleaning and painting. Everyone working on old houses should take at least a one-day lead awareness course. **F** (state contacts)

19

- Some work should only be done by a person with professional training. **F** This includes:
  - Preparing large, damaged lead-painted surfaces for painting (like the side of a house).
  - Removing moldings that expose cavities like window jambs or baseboards.
  - Stripping on-site using chemicals.
  - Demolishing known or potentially lead-painted surfaces.

Responsibilities of Landlords & Renters

Landlords sometimes claim that lead paint was there before they owned the property, or they were told to use lead paint, therefore, the presence of lead paint is not their fault. This may be so, but a risk from lead paint is usually because of poor maintenance, not just because lead paint is present. Therefore, it is the responsibility of the property owner.

Landlord Responsibilities

The Title X Task Force ②, which was set up to develop national lead policy, has outlined the responsibilities of property owners for maintenance and standards of care. **E**

- A house or apartment should be free from defects that cause water damage (see Chapter 2). Defects causing water or moisture damage are also housing code violations.

Plaster that is kept dry and maintained can last a long time without ever having to be re-plastered.

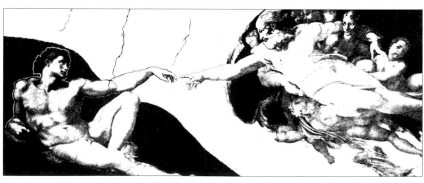

Plaster ceiling of the Sistine Chapel, Michelangelo Buonarroti 1510

- All painted surfaces should be sound and free of flaking and peeling paint. In most places this is also a housing code requirement.
- Horizontal surfaces—floors, steps, window stools and troughs—should be smooth and cleanable.
- Doors and windows should be free of abrasion that rubs through paint layers or crushes painted surfaces.
- Windows, doors, walls, ceilings and floors should be structurally sound.
- Property owners should have wall-to-wall carpet cleaned as needed. It is preferable to have it removed and replaced with area rugs and/or hall and staircase runners.③
- Property owners should have a "third party" (a professional not related to them) dust test before a new tenant moves in. Test results should be under the clearance levels set by HUD. **A** This record can also help protect the property owner from being successfully sued, as long as he/she maintains the property.
- If there is any evidence of children chewing on painted surfaces, the property owner should determine if the surface is painted with lead. If so, the paint must be enclosed, encapsulated or removed (not chemically stripped, as this does not remove all lead—see Chapter 5).

It is against the law for a property owner to evict, harass, or threaten a tenants because they have complained about a housing condition.

Renter Responsibilities

- It is the responsibility of occupants to clean their own homes, but cleaning up lead dust requires special cleaning. Lead-painted surfaces must be well maintained for cleaning to be effective.
- Occupants should inform the property owner at the first sign of water damage or flaking paint.
- Occupants should keep clothes off floors as much as possible and clean rugs or send them to cleaners.

Work Principles

There are certain principles which should be observed whether someone is working on their own home or a professional is doing the work. (Do not assume a person calling him/herself "a professional" knows more than you.)

- **Create as little dust as possible.**
  Avoid demolition where possible. Do not use power tools on leaded surfaces, particularly power sanders.

- **If the work releases any dust, keep it damp.**
  Mist work surfaces with a misting bottle as you scrape flaking paint or clean up paint chips. When removing molding, cut painted joints with a utility knife and mist surfaces before removal.

- **Keep dust contained.**
  Where possible, keep doors and windows closed to prevent dust from blowing. Work over a plastic drop cloth. Wear shoe covers and remove them or remove shoes if you step off drop cloth. Isolate the work area from the rest of the house. **C**

- **Clean up as you work.**
  Even though the entire house will be cleaned at the end of the job, clean up each work area as you go.

- **Keep all children out of work area.**
  When minor work is done, do a complete clean-up **B** and take dust samples **A** before allowing children back into the work area.

> **If large amounts of dust are created by the work, wait until your lead test results are reported from the lab and show clearance levels have been achieved before you re-occupy the house.**

Prevention is the Key

Whether or not you know if paint in your house contains lead, assume that it does unless your house was built after 1978, or you have had it tested and found no lead. **Remember, intact lead paint does not pose a hazard.** Protective maintenance is critical. 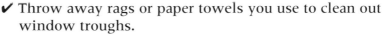 If you find high dust levels, at least clean up the dust. Try to discover the source and correct the problem.

Fix

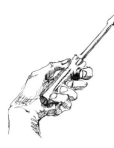

Repairing the causes of paint failure that create lead dust is the first step.
- ✔ Fix sources of moisture such as a leaky roof.
- ✔ Repair gutters and downspouts.
- ✔ Adjust doors so they don't scrape.
- ✔ Cover impact surfaces such as outside corners.
- ✔ Make surfaces smooth and cleanable.

Clean

Damp cleaning the house is important for keeping dust levels low.
- ✔ Throw away rags or paper towels you use to clean out window troughs.
- ✔ Use a string mop and a mop squeezer. Change mop heads often.
- ✔ Professionally clean carpet. (However, even professionally cleaned carpets can still contain lead dust. ③)
- ✔ Clean children's toys, pacifiers, etc. often.

Maintain

- ✔ Keep all painted surfaces intact. Prevent paint chipping by protecting wall and trim edges. To prepare for painting, wet scrape or wet sand. If paint peels, find and repair the cause.
- ✔ Keep gutters and downspouts clean and in good condition.
- ✔ Vent moisture from bathroom and kitchen; keep basements and crawl spaces dry.
- ✔ Keep wood windows and doors adjusted and in good working order.

Monitor

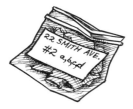

- ✔ If you have found a lead hazard and addressed what seems to be the cause, you should continue to monitor dust (and possibly soil and water) to be sure the hazard does not return. **A**

Stabilize, Clean and Maintain

In all cases, take children out of the house during work that may disturb lead paint. They should not return before final clean-up is complete.

If work has created much dust, children should not return until dust samples are taken and results show clearance levels have been achieved.

Cleaning and Stabilizing

Following are the work procedures for stabilizing a small area of paint that is flaking, chipping, or showing signs of friction. If caution is used, and only small amounts of dust are created and then immediately cleaned up, a homeowner can safely do this work.

- Remove all rugs, drapes, spreads, etc. near the work area and send to the cleaners. Move furniture away from the work area. Wall-to-wall carpeting and upholstered furniture near work area should be covered with plastic. Remove objects from furniture and remove all children's toys and furniture from the room. Wipe them with a "tack cloth" (you can buy these in hardware stores).

- Attach plastic to the baseboards under the work area with duct tape or masking tape (6 mil plastic is best **F**). Extend the plastic 5 feet in all directions from the work area. Have all tools and supplies at the work area before work begins.

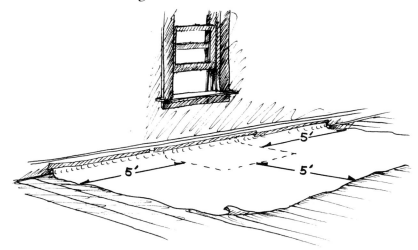

- Avoid tracking dust by removing work shoes when stepping off plastic, or wear "paper" throwaway booties over shoes **F** on the drop cloth, and remove them each time you step off the drop cloth. Close door to room and keep windows closed to avoid a draft blowing dust off the plastic. Turn off forced air system.

Stabilize, Clean and Maintain

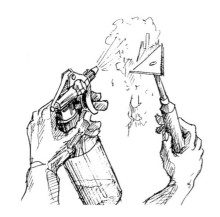

Always mist work area as you work to keep down dust.

• Where small amounts of paint are flaking or there is a ridge of paint where molding has been removed, mist the area with water and gently scrape off the loose paint.

• This area can then be lightly sanded with a wet abrasive sponge (these can be purchased at a hardware store). Keep dipping the sponge in a pail of water as you work to clean the sponge and keep down dust.

• When small amounts of wet scraping are completed, smooth rough areas of wall with a skim coat of spackle. Wood can be smoothed with wood filler. After these dry, lightly wet sand with a wet abrasive sponge or wet wet/dry sandpaper. Clean, and where necessary, degrease entire surface. Prime with best-grade primer and repaint. If paint is glossy, degloss with "liquid sandpaper" or a wet abrasive sponge.

• Special products, like encapsulants, can be used in small areas to cover or stabilize paint. (See Chapter 5 for details.)

The Title X Task Force developed a report, <u>Putting the Pieces Together</u>, that outlines recommendations for national policy. **F** Within the report is a proposal for minimum maintenance practices of occupied units and standard treatments to be done at turn-over (between occupants) for pre-1950 units. **E**

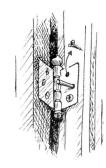

Door Work

When a door is rubbing against the jamb on the latch side, the hinge screws may be loose. To check for loose hinges, open the door, hold both door knobs and try to move the door up and down. If it moves up and down, hinge screws are loose and need to be tightened. If screws are stripped, remove them one at a time. Put a dowel in the hole, break or cut it off flush with the surface of the hinge leaf and screw a new phillips-head screw into the dowel or install a screw ½" longer than the original screw.

• If door is crushing against the jamb on the hinge side or scraping against the latch-side jamb or head jamb after screws are tightened, pull hinge pins and remove hinge leaves from door. If the door is crushing on the hinge side and there is space on the latch side, try putting a few shims under the hinge leaf. If this makes the door scrape against the jamb on the latch side, mist the hinge-side edge of the door and hand plane the surface until there is clearance on both sides when the door is rehung. This must be done on a plastic drop cloth. Lay the door on its latch edge to plane its hinge edge. The only wood-to-wood contact should be the face of the door against the door-stop molding on the latch side. (The face of the hinge leaves should be above the surgface of the door edge.)

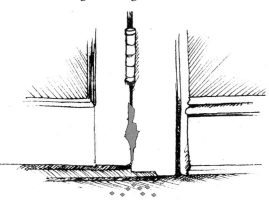

A loose top hinge, swollen door, or poorly hung door causes crushing along this edge.

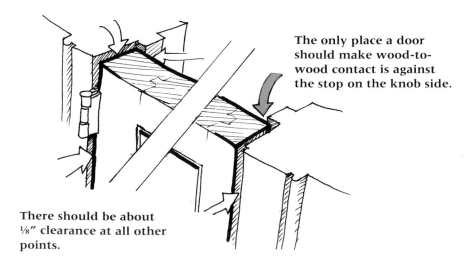

The only place a door should make wood-to-wood contact is against the stop on the knob side.

There should be about ⅛" clearance at all other points.

Windows

Remove the inside stop and wet scrape the ridges of paint left on the sash and jamb, then replace with a new stop.

- Drill two holes (1/4") at the bottom of the storm window frame to let water out. The holes need to be flush with the sill.
- Clean out trough. Cut a piece of aluminum flashing to fit trough. The flashing can be scored with a utility knife then bent back and forth or cut with tin snips. Caulk around the back face of the flashing, lay in trough in bed of adhesive caulk. Then caulk the perimeter around the top edge. This leaves the trough clean and cleanable. It looks better to use white flashing. You may notch the flashing around the moldings or drive a chisel under the bottom of the moldings so the flashing can slide under them against the jamb.
- Wet scrape and repaint exterior.

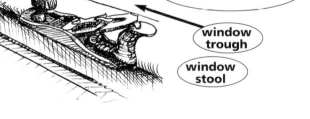

- Mist the leading edge of the window stool. Plane the edge down to clean wood. Plane as much surface on bottom and top as the plane can reach. A couple of inches in from the edge is enough. Small amounts of paint remaining in corners can be wet scraped. Then wet sand the wood, prime and paint. This operation makes the surface lead-free. This work is not necessary if paint on the stool is in good shape and there is no evidence of a child chewing on the edge.

In many cases it is more cost-effective to replace windows. Replacement windows lower energy and maintenance costs and add value to the house, as well as address a major lead hazard.

Clean, Test and Maintain

Clean each area as you work, then clean the entire house before children return. It is important that the cleaning be done properly. **B**

- Take a dust sample in the work area, but also do a composite test in a few other areas to be sure dust has not spread. **A**
- Remember, the effectiveness of this work is based on how well the house is maintained; roof flashing, gutters and downspouts must be kept in good condition. All painted surfaces must be kept intact and cleanable.

Soil Around the House

Bare soil that has become contaminated by lead from paint chips, particularly where children play, can be a hazard. Test the soil around your house. **A**

Where children play in bare soil and the levels are 400 to 2,000 parts per million:

- Move play equipment away from bare soil.
- Restrict children's access to bare soil.
- Prevent further contamination of area by stabilizing paint on exterior surfaces.

If the levels are over 2,000 parts per million, cover the soil with grass or sod. Planting shrubs next to house is particularly helpful, as this is usually an area with high lead levels. The ground can be covered with wood chips or gravel. Wood chips also hold moisture and protect shrubbery from dry weather and cold.

If the levels are over 5,000 parts per million, a thin layer of soil may need to be removed, or a permanent cover like concrete can be installed. This should be done by professionals.

Holistic Intervention

A cost-effective and health-based approach to maintaining a home must be holistic (the view that an organic or integrated whole has a reality independent of and greater than the sum of its parts. WEBSTER).

- Enclosing exterior walls with vinyl or aluminum siding that is not properly vented can increase the degradation of interior paint, destroy insulation, and rot the structure of a house. (Cover old siding with Tyvek® before enclosing with vented siding.)
- Wall-to-wall carpets can hold large amounts of lead dust, encourage mold growth—thereby increasing respiratory disease, and hold food particles which encourage roach infestation. (Seal wood floors, then replace wall-to-wall carpets with area rugs and runners. ③)
- Sealing up the house too tightly can increase carbon monoxide, radon and other airborne contaminants, and can increase mold and mildew (a bathroom exhaust fan is part of the solution).

Beginning an environmental audit with an energy audit is recommended. The auditor should look for moisture problems, make sure there are sufficient air changes and sufficient "make-up air" for combustion units such as furnaces and hot water heaters. This is particularly important before a renovation.

An effective plan looks at the relationship among weatherization, lead paint, carbon monoxide, microbe growth, dry rot, roaches, and air quality. Few professionals have the ability to take into account these related factors. But an informed home owner can buy carbon monoxide and radon detectors, replace wall-to-wall carpeting with area rugs, keep the house vented while still saving energy, and maintain the roof and window systems.

Notes

Chapter 4

If evaluating your situation and/or doing the work yourself is not something you can do properly or safely, consider hiring a professional.

There are four general areas of responsibility:
- Determining the risk and its causes
- Designing and pricing the work
- Doing the work safely
- Making sure the work was done right

This work can be done by any combination of professionals, but if you are hiring someone to do the work, a "third party"— a person unrelated to the person doing the work—should do the final test—the clearance test.

Where there is a poisoned child or government funding is involved, specific certifications for particular jobs may be required. In unregulated situations, you have the following options:

Effective professionals can answer all these questions:

What's the problem?

Do we have a problem that will make anyone in my family sick?

How bad is it?

What caused it and how can I fix the cause?

What needs to be done?

How do we prioritize the proposed work, given a limited budget?

Who should do the work?

   (They may choose not to recommend a contractor, but you should still be able to request a list of people they believe are qualified.)

Do we need to move out during work? If not, how will we be kept safe?

How do we know if someone we hire is doing it right?

How long will it take?

What work might we do ourselves?

Inspection and Risk Assessment

Inspection

An inspection without a risk assessment only tells you the lead content of every painted surface. Remember, the mere presence of lead may not present a risk. An inspector uses an

XRF machine for this measurement. **A** This person must be certified in most states.

An inspection is useful if:

- It is part of a risk assessment.
- You want to determine if a house is "lead-free."
- You intend to demolish several painted surfaces and you want to determine the risk from lead.

Risk Assessment

A risk assessment should give you most of the information you will need to make decisions, including:

- Is there lead in any failing paint? (A chip test or XRF may be used.)
- Are there high levels of lead in household dust, your water system or exterior soil?
- If problems are found, what are the probable causes? What are the best solutions?

In most states a risk assessor must be certified (this certification usually includes an inspector's certification). However, unless a certified risk assessor has extensive experience as a housing inspector, contractor or tradesperson, it is unlikely he or she will be skilled at determining what work needs to be done. A person who has extensive housing experience and has taken a lead paint supervisors course may be capable of performing a risk survey that includes the visual survey interview and samples as described in Chapter 2. (Anyone can take the two-day risk assessor course, but in most states, they can not become a certified risk assessor without first being certified as an inspector.)

As solving lead problems is a new craft, few companies have sufficient training or experience. So, if you hire a "professional," it is important that both you and they have an understanding of safe work practices, clean-up procedures and clearance techniques.

A contractor may be certified with only four days of training. To be effective, a contractor needs both training and experience. DO NOT ASSUME A CONTRACTOR KNOWS MORE THAN YOU.

BEWARE!

The professional who tries to panic you into doing more than you need to do.

The tradesperson who denies there is a risk. "I've been tearing out lead paint my whole life and there's nothing wrong with me..."

The professional who doesn't explain things because "it's too complicated for you to understand."

The Contractor's Responsibility

The contractor doing the work is responsible for:
- Writing a contract that includes a specification of work and an agreed cost.
- Doing the work on time and in a "workperson-like" manner.
- Protecting an occupant's health and safety.
- Keeping workers safe.
- Protecting your home, both the work area and the rest of your home.
- Protecting the neighborhood and the environment.
- Passing a dust clearance test at the end of a job that may produce lead dust. It is recommended that you don't make final payment until you have third-party clearance results back. You can do the dust tests yourself, but they don't carry the legal weight of third-party tests.

Hiring a Contractor

A poorly trained contractor doing renovations or preparation of lead-painted surfaces can poison his or her own workers as well as the residence if the work is not done correctly and cleaned up to the highest standards. (Again assume all paint on pre-1978 houses is lead unless a test shows it is not.)

QUESTIONS TO ASK THE CONTRACTOR
Is the Contractor...

Licensed?

Checking on a license can also reveal if there have been unresolved complaints. Not all states have contractor licensing. Check local regulations. **F**

Insured?

✔ Worker's Compensation, in case a worker gets hurt on the job.

✔ Liability, in case someone else gets injured on the job.

✔ Property insurance, in case the property gets damaged (some contractors may also have special lead insurance, but this is not necessary).

Recommended?

Ask the contractor for a list of recently completed jobs and phone numbers, so you can choose from the list to check references. This is <u>extremely</u> important.

Trained?

All workers who break or disturb lead-painted surfaces—maintenance workers, painters, window installers, weatherization workers, etc.—should take at least a one-day awareness training. Unfortunately, a one-day training is not available in many states. Call your state information contact to see what training is available. **F**

Doing work poorly can be more dangerous than not doing any work!

All work breaking lead-painted surfaces is lead work!

Hiring a Professional

Certified?
Check local and state regulations to see if contractors, site supervisors and/or workers need certification.

Skilled?
Be sure the person you are hiring is a dependable business person and a skilled craftsperson. Do not assume a person with a few days training and/or certification is skilled. It is critical that someone who has years of renovation experience be directly supervising the work.

Informed?
The major guidance document for lead work is the *HUD Lead Based Paint Guidelines*. The contractor should be familiar with this document. You can purchase this document by calling 1-800-245-2691. Ask the contractor what his or her plans are for:
- Containment
- Clean-Up
- Worker Protection
- Disposal

It is strongly recommended, and in some states required by law, **F** that workers doing substantial renovation and/or lead hazard abatement take the EPA lead workers' course. This course runs from one to four days and is available throughout the country. Where workers are doing low-risk work not requiring certification, and a one-day training course is not available, this book may provide sufficient information to keep workers and occupants safe.

Supervisors running jobs that break or disturb painted surfaces on old houses are urged to take an EPA supervisors training regardless of state requirements.

Developing a Scope of Work

The scope of work is a description of the work to be done. If you hire a risk assessor, he/she will develop a scope of work. A contractor can also develop a scope of work. This can be written so you can choose items within your budget prioritized by their urgency. This can be done without revealing your budget. Ask the contractor to organize work in three categories using the following form. You can then "draw the line" where the cost of work uses up the budget.

URGENT TASKS
Those tasks which must be done
for the safety of children. (If not done,
it is recommended that the children
be removed from the house.)   Total Cost $ _____

PRIORITY TASKS   Item $ _____
Other critical tasks in order of importance.   Item $ _____

LONG-TERM MAINTENANCE   Item $ _____
Those items that should be done   Item $ _____
in the near future, like repair or   Item $ _____
replace roof, insulate attic, etc.   Item $ _____

Writing a Contract

Don't sign something you don't understand or don't like. A clear contract is good for both the contractor and the customer.

In lead work the final product is important, but so is how the job gets done!

Any contract should include:

Your right to cancel within 3 days.

Duration—How long an estimated price will be honored. How long job will take. How soon it will start. By what date will it end.

Warranties—Appliances, roofs, windows, etc., should have a warranty. You should receive copies of warranties before you make final payment. Each one should include the name of the company, the address, how long the warranty is for and what is covered.

Payments—A payment schedule should include a draw schedule with no more than 1/3 down. ④
The contract should spell out what work is to be completed before each payment. Hold out at least 10% until after completion, when clearance results are received.

Specifications—
- They should define what work is to be done and where.
- They should prescribe model and brand of special orders. (Ask to sign samples of chosen colors, textures and styles, such as tile patterns or special molding.)

All contracts that call for breaking many surfaces of old, painted wood (unless tested to prove there is no lead paint) should include:

1. **Worker Protection.**
   This should include respirators and protective clothing during dusty work.
2. **Isolating Living Space.**
   If anyone is living in a building where work will create large amounts of lead dust, like demolition or large amounts of paint scraping, the work area must be totally sealed from the living space. **C** The seal must not be broken until final clean-up **B** and successful clearance dust test results are received. **A** (Entrance to the space would be through an exterior door or window.)
3. **Clearance Clean-Up.**
   The contract must commit to a clean-up using correct procedures. You may include information from Appendix **B** in the contract.
4. **Clearance Test.**
   The contract should include a provision that the final payment will not be made until final dust clearance is achieved. **A** It is better if the property owner hires a person to do the clearance test who has no relation to the contractor. This is a "third-party" person. The clearance test may cost between $50 and $150. **F**

The Cost

If lead paint work is done, as it should be, as part of other work, there is no reason for it to add a great deal of cost.

Costs vary too much to present specific numbers, but a contractor who understands how to integrate lead work into regular maintenance or rehab will be able to do the job for a small percent more than non-lead work.

It has been estimated that doing a lead-sensitive turnover treatment or renovation will increase the total cost by no more than 15 to 25%.

Notes

Chapter 5

Whether you hire a professional or do the work yourself, you should understand all aspects of the work.

If you choose to do the the work yourself, attend at least a one-day awareness training. If such a training is not available, this chapter will outline key work practices.

This chapter is designed for people who already have carpentry skills. It discusses how you can do some of your own work but does not give detailed directions for each procedure.

Levels of Risk and Safe Work Practices

Various levels of work carry different levels of risk to occupants and workers. On large jobs, professionals may determine the risk by air monitoring, which involves taking a sample to measure what level of airborne dust a particular work practice may generate. ⑤

In all cases it is recommended that the work area receive a complete clean-up. If there is a possibility of increased lead dust, do a dust wipe test after clean-up. **A**

The following are guidelines for various work practices. They are valuable but can not guarantee the safety of workers or occupants. For safe lead work practices in low-risk situations, please see Chapter 3.

The practices are divided into three levels of risk:

Very Low Risk

Work that creates very little dust in a small area of the home. This would include maintenance practices such as spot painting or wall repair of a few square feet, repairing a window, and rehanging a door.

Occupancy - The work area should be closed off. Children should not enter the area until clean-up is complete.

Masking - Protect the floor around the work area with a poly drop cloth taped to the baseboard. See Chapter 3 for step-by-step instructions. Clean the drop cloth before moving it.

Worker Protection - Workers should wear a dust mask for minimum protection and booties when on the drop cloth, to avoid tracking debris, paint, caulk, etc. off the drop cloth. (Workers may also change shoes or damp wipe their shoes upon leaving the work area.)

Work Practices

 Moderate Risk
Work that creates small amounts of dust.

Occupancy - Children should be out of the apartment or home until the work is complete and final clean-up is done unless the work area is completely isolated from the living space.

Masking - Extend a poly drop cloth five feet from work area. Tape edge against wall to baseboard (see p. 24). If work will be done to entire room, such as wet scraping all walls in preparation for painting, or there is wall-to-wall carpeting, cover the entire floor with poly, and duct tape it to the baseboard.

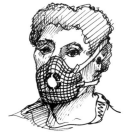

Worker wearing NIOSH-approved dust mask.

Worker Protection - Workers should wear NIOSH-approved dust masks. It says this on the mask package. They should wear shoe covers and remove them or their shoes when leaving the work area. Clothing should be changed or vacuumed upon leaving the work area. Clothing can also be protected by disposable Tyvek® coveralls to be removed upon leaving the work area.

 High Risk
Work that creates a large amount of dust. This work includes:

- Tearing open or removing a plaster wall.
- Demolishing door jambs and casing, or ripping out window jambs (removing just the window sash creates very little dust).
- Chemical stripping of paint on site (this work should be avoided unless workers have specific training).
- Removing old wallpaper that may be painted with lead paint.
- Wet scraping large areas of flaking or peeling paint, like the side of a house or several rooms.

Occupancy - All children and unprotected adults must stay out of the work area until final clean-up and dust test results are received indicating levels are below clearance. Post a sign at entrance that says: LEAD HAZARD; NO SMOKING, EATING OR DRINKING.

Masking - Work area must be completely isolated from living space. ◲ Seal is not to be broken until dust clearance has been achieved.

Work Practices

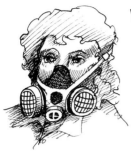

Worker wearing
a respirator.

Worker Protection -
- •Workers must wear respirators, which should be fit tested (this may be done where they are purchased).
- • Tyvek suits should be worn, and where possible, workers should change and shower before going home. At least vacuum clothing.
- • Booties must be worn in dirty area or shoes changed.
- • Wear goggles to protect eyes.
- • Wear a painter's cap or hood to protect hair.

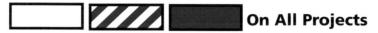 **On All Projects**

- • Wash hands and face before leaving work area.
- • Clean work area at end of job. **B**
- • Do dust tests to be sure cleaning was done properly. **A** On low or moderate-risk jobs where little dust is created and complete clean-up is done, waiting for results would not be necessary before re-occupancy. (State and local regulations should always be checked.)

Disposal - Disposal of construction rubbish which may contain lead is subject to local regulations. Following are recommended, and prudent, practices:
- • Small amounts of trash produced by home owners working in their own homes can be put out with the garbage. Wash water can be dumped into the toilet (do not use sinks or dump outside). Home owners usually fall under a "residential exclusion," which means they do not need to determine whether their waste is hazardous.
- • In all cases waste that may contain lead should be wrapped in poly and taped or sealed in garbage bags, and kept away from children.
- • Contractors should send all construction waste to a rubble land fill, never to an incinerator. This includes poly drop cloths, window sashes, old doors, etc. In most areas if less than 220 pounds of lead paint waste is created in one month, the contractor is considered by the EPA to be a "conditionally exempt small quantity generator" and does not need to determine if the waste is hazardous waste.
- • The liquid that is generated by water-blasting paint off a building's exterior, or the goo from stripping large areas of a house's exterior, are exceptions. These <u>must</u> be contained and tested to determine if the waste is required to go to a hazardous waste facility. (This is one reason these removal techniques are strongly discouraged. They are dangerous and expensive.)

Terms

Before discussing specific treatments of parts of a house, here are some definitions:

> **Abatement -** A measure that will protect occupants for at least 20 years.
>
> **Hazard Abatement -** Abating only specific surfaces and edges that might present a hazard, or do so already.
>
> **Abatement Techniques -** There are four types of abatement techniques:

ENCLOSURE

This involves putting a hard surface, like dry wall, paneling, wainscot, etc. over a lead-painted surface. This provides an excellent barrier. It must be mechanically fastened to the ceiling joists, wall studs, or wood substrate. It must also be caulked or otherwise sealed along its perimeter. This is particularly important at the base of walls, where lead dust can fall down behind the enclosure and drift out the bottom. The caulking should be done on the rear perimeter.

ENCAPSULATION

Encapsulants are special paints that are brushed, rolled, sprayed or troweled on.

Encapsulants are particularly good for walls where the plaster or wood is sound and there is not a great deal of paint de-lamination. Where there is some de-lamination of paint surfaces but the plaster or wood substrate (the painted material) is intact, a mesh system can be used. Encapsulants should be tested on a surface that represents the area in the poorest condition that you intend to encapsulate. There are some elaborate testing methods, but the basic principle is, test to ensure that the encapsulant cannot be easily scraped off the underlying surface.

REMOVAL AND REPLACEMENT

With one exception, the only method that creates a lead-<u>free</u> surface is removing the building component and replacing it. (The exception is removing both the paint and the very top layer of wood with a hand plane.) Removing a baseboard, window or door, casing or jambs can release a great deal of dust and should be done in an isolated area. Workers should wear respiratory protection. HEPA vacuum behind baseboards or window casing as soon as they are removed to eliminate accumulated dust.

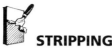 **STRIPPING**

On-site chemical stripping is expensive and dangerous. It should only be done by a trained and experienced professional. The goo that takes off the paint can get into cracks, and days later dry and turn to dust, creating an increased hazard. It can severely burn a worker's eyes or skin. If not well neutralized and cleaned up it can burn the new paint. There are some strippers that are less dangerous, but they tend to not strip as well. Never use strippers containing methylene chloride, which has been shown to cause cancer.

Off-site chemical stripping is safer, but even off-site stripped wood still contains lead in the top layer. For this reason it should not be belt sanded, and is not safe for easily chewable surfaces.

Mechanical stripping with hand, not power tools, is the safest stripping technique. An example is using a hand plane after misting the work surface, to remove paint from the edge of a window stool or the hinge edge of a door. A HEPA sander may also be used. ⑨

Work Practices by Building Component

The following practices are more likely to be necessary where maintenance has been deferred. They are usually combined with the stabilization techniques discussed in Chapter 3. These practices are more permanent and more expensive, but since they will last longer, they may be less expensive over time. Most take a higher level of skill.

These symbols are used in the rest of the chapter to categorize the various practices by level of risk and work technique.

☐ **Very Low Risk**   ▨ **Moderate Risk**   ■ **High Risk**

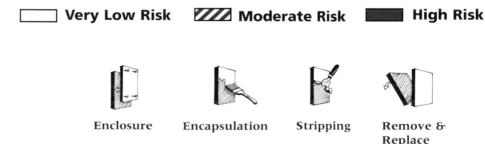

Enclosure   Encapsulation   Stripping   Remove & Replace

Complete removal and replacement of an architectural component is always an option, but it is expensive, may create a hazard, and may destroy architectural detail.

WINDOWS

Restoration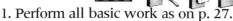

1. Perform all basic work as on p. 27.
2. Remove inside stop and bottom sash. Be careful to tie off counter-weight rope so you can re-attach the counter weights. If top sash is in poor condition and will be raised and lowered, remove it and the parting bead and treat it the same as bottom sash. It saves labor to fix top sash in place and wet scrape and repaint it as part of exterior work.
3. Wet scrape and/or mist and hand plane friction edges of sash. Wet scrape, wet sand, prime and paint sash before reinstalling.
4. Wet scrape and prime jamb as necessary.
5. Repair counter-weight system as necessary. Replace cord with chain or install some system to safely keep the sash in a raised position. (Never prop open a window with a stick, as a child moving the stick may be seriously injured.)
6. Re-install prepared or new sash into opening. Install new stop. You can also install vinyl compression track. (This approach is good for historic preservation, but is labor-intensive and may be more expensive than a vinyl replacement window).
   Vinyl compression track **F** can be cut with a plexiglass cutter so only the bottom sash is in channel. The top sash would be fixed in place.

Diagram labels: casing, top sash, jamb (extends to outside), bottom sash, inside stop, outside stop, trough, parting bead, sill, stool, apron

Replacement Window

1. Remove stop, bead and sash as above.
2. Install vinyl replacement window against outside stop in a bead of caulk. (If outside stop is in poor condition, replace.) Or install new, wood double-glazed sash into tracks that allow for tilt in.

Complete Window Replacement

1. Remove window sash, casing, stool, apron and jamb. Sill may be saved or replaced. It is recommended this be done by a manufacturer's representative, but they probably will not be trained in lead work and this is a dusty job. Be sure the worksite is isolated from living space and not opened until complete clean-up is finished. **C**

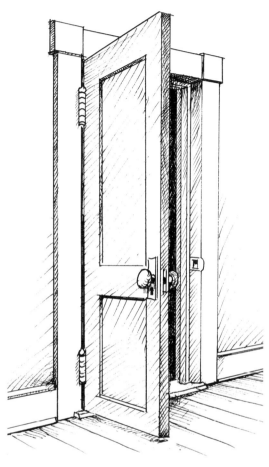

DOORS

Restoration

To save an original panel door with paint in condition too poor to simply treat on site:

1. Remove hinge pins and send door to a stripper. When door returns, paint pigment will be gone but lead will remain in grain. If door needs sanding, room must be completely isolated **C** and respirator must be worn. It may be easier to fill, wet sand, and repaint.

2. Unless jamb is in poor shape, simply wet scrape and repaint (same for casing). If casing is in poor shape it is easiest to replace with similar pattern. If historic value requires off-site stripping and re-installation, it may be easier to repaint than to stain.

3. If jamb is in poor shape it may be necessary to strip on site. This is better done by a professional. It is much easier to replace the stop molding, or if it is a rabbeted jamb, use a rabbet plane to remove paint on contact edge or wet scrape.

Replacement

1. In most cases it is easiest to remove an old door and casing and install a new, pre-hung flush or panel door in the original door jamb, as long as this doesn't make opening too small.

2. New casing works better if it is wider than the old casing by several inches to cover up old damaged wall. You may need to purchase ogee or bead edge baseboard if the casing that is available is too narrow. Caulk back perimeter of casing before installing to keep dust from escaping.

FLOORS

Where a floor is painted with lead paint, it will represent a hazard as it will be constantly abraded by moving furniture and foot traffic.

An interim control measure is to seal the floor with a high-grade deck paint or other sealer, cover walkways with runners and area rugs, and put protective rubber cups under furniture legs.

Enclosure

A permanent solution is to cover floor with a good grade plywood (exterior glued for bathroom and kitchen). Then install tile, vinyl, parquet, etc. The floor could also be covered with tongue-and-groove flooring.

There may be sanding machines for rent with HEPA vac attached, but they are difficult to find. Even with a HEPA vac, respiratory protection, complete isolation of the work area, and extreme care are recommended.

STAIRCASES

Staircases are consistently abraded and chipped from traffic. An interim control measure is a carpet runner on the traffic area.

Enclosure

A permanent solution is to enclose treads and risers. A metal nose on the tread lasts much longer than a rubber tread with a rubber nose.

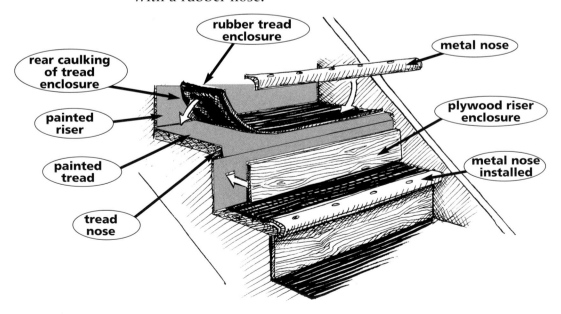

rubber tread enclosure

metal nose

rear caulking of tread enclosure

painted riser

plywood riser enclosure

painted tread

metal nose installed

tread nose

WALLS AND CEILINGS

Encapsulants

Walls are usually not painted with lead-based paint. Bathrooms and kitchen walls are most likely to have lead paint. You may send in a chip sample **A** before doing extensive work on a wall.

Where walls are in poor condition and paint is beginning to flake, crack, or "alligator" but is not de-laminating in large areas, and the substrate (plaster or wood) is sound, encapsulants can be effective. One product that has been used for several decades is Glid-Wall,® distributed by the Glidden Paint Company. A coating gets rolled on, a mesh goes on and a second coat gets rolled over the mesh. Other encapsulants are mentioned on the resource sheet. **F** Before applying encapsulants, the wall should be cleaned and wet scraped just as one would prep for painting. If this results in some paint flaking off several layers down, it should be presumed to be lead paint and extra care should be taken with masking and clean-up.

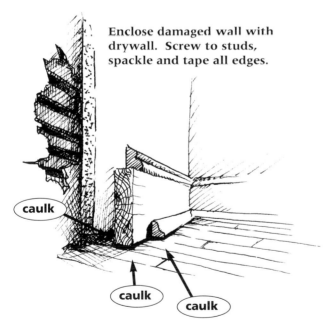

Enclose damaged wall with drywall. Screw to studs, spackle and tape all edges.

caulk

caulk

caulk

Enclosure

Enclosing a surface involves mechanically fastening dry wall, wood, metal, etc. to the surface. It is a safe and very long-lasting solution.

Enclosing a wall or ceiling will increase the degradation of paint on the enclosed wall. It is therefore critical to seal the perimeter, particularly the bottom of a wall (see illustration). Drop ceilings and wallpaper are not enclosures.

Precautions during enclosing:
- HEPA vac bottom of old wall at floor
- Spray fine dusting of boric acid under wall before installing baseboard to discourage roaches.
- Set baseboard then shoe molding into a bead of twenty-year-plus caulk to seal bottom of wall.

EXTERIOR WALLS

Exterior walls are the most problematic surface of a house because of their large area, inaccessibility, and the probability of paint damage.

Damage to outside paint is a natural effect of sun and weather, but moisture from inside the house can greatly accelerate the damage to exterior paint.

If the paint is in fairly good condition it will probably be least expensive to wet scrape and paint. This may not be the most cost-effective over time. Wet scraping and repainting is not abatement, but may stabilize the paint.

Wet Scraping and Repainting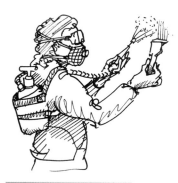

Risk is determined by surface area and amount of loose paint. Remember, you are only removing <u>loose</u> paint, not removing paint down to the brick or wood.

1. Set up 6 mil poly drop cloths 10 feet out from house and 5 feet more for each additional story on which you are working. Do not work outside if there is enough wind to blow chips and dust past or off plastic. It helps to turn up edges of plastic. Don't use booties on ladders. Never put a leaning ladder on plastic. Cut through plastic for ladder feet, then patch holes with duct tape. **D**

2. Mist a few feet at a time as you scrape, keeping the area you are scraping damp. (A small pump sprayer carried in a knapsack is very convenient.) Do not hose down wall as it will spread paint chips. Clean surface before painting.

3. Be sure windows are closed in work area and then well cleaned. The house should be entered by the door furthest from the work area so as to avoid tracking in lead dust.

4. The paint job is only as good as the primer. Buy the best primer and use paint designed to go with the primer. Most paint companies sell special primer that grips old paint. Where wood is exposed, use wood sealer first.

Encapsulant paints are more expensive but may be cheaper over time, as they last longer. **F**

Uncontained sanding, grinding or power washing exterior paint can generate toxic levels of lead in the immediate neighborhood which can travel through open windows.

Enclosure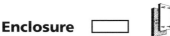

Covering wood siding with aluminum or vinyl can create moisture problems behind the new siding and may do long-term damage to the house. It is therefore very important that the new siding be well vented. To contain the old lead paint and cut down on air infiltration, first cover the wall with building paper . This will allow moisture to leave the wall cavity and act as a drainage plane.

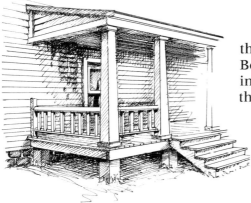

PORCHES

Because porches are exposed to weather, they tend to suffer extensive paint damage. Before doing work on a porch be sure the flashing, where the porch roof meets the house, and the roof are in good shape.

The following suggestions are only for cases where the paint is in such poor shape that wet scraping and re-painting are not sufficient. If the wood is rotted it must be replaced before any other work is done.

Ceiling

Enclose with an exterior plywood like Texture 1-11. Back caulk the perimeter to seal before installing.

Posts

There are some encapsulants designed for exterior application that would work well. **F**

Balustrades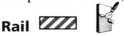

If in moderately poor shape, try an encapsulant. If in very poor shape it is usually easier to remove and replace them.

Rail

As this is a "mouthable" surface, mechanically stripping is advisable. Using a hand plane is safe and inexpensive.

Floor/Steps

If the floor or steps are painted with lead paint they will need to be replaced or enclosed. See p. 46. (Floor sanders with HEPA vacs attached may be available.)

For More Information

See HUD Guidelines described on Resource page 82. **F**

Eight Things to Remember

1 There are affordable prevention solutions.

2 Lead paint poisoning can do serious permanent damage, particularly to children.

3 Most poisoning is due to dust from failing paint, so use dust tests to measure risks.

4 Lead paint, if maintained, may pose no threat.

5 The best and cheapest time to address lead paint is as part of maintenance, during turnover from one occupant to another and during renovation.

6 Removing lead paint in a way that turns it to dust may be far more dangerous than leaving it alone.

7 There are many problems in homes that can make occupants, particularly children, sick. They include carbon monoxide, lead dust, roaches, mold, cold drafts, a lack of ventilation, dust mites, insecticides, etc. Many are caused by moisture. They can best be dealt with as a whole.

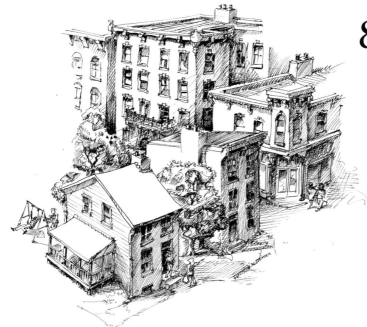

8 Lead poisoning and other indoor environmental problems can best be solved by the people already doing work on the house—property owners, maintenance workers, renovators, homeowners, and community housing organizations. They do need some training, however, and hopefully this book will help.

Testing is critical when you want to know:

- **Is there a risk?**
- **What work do we need to do?**
- **Was it cleaned properly?**
- **Has the risk returned?**

There are two categories of testing.

1. Tests that determine if there is a <u>risk</u> of lead-paint poisoning.

2. Tests that determine if lead paint is present on a particular surface.

Some tests do both.

Tests to Determine a <u>Risk of Lead Poisoning.</u>

<u>Peeling Paint</u> If an XRF, chip or chemical test is done on a surface where paint is peeling, these tests also determine risk.

<u>Dust</u> This test takes samples of house dust to determine how much lead is in the dust. The sample is sent to a lab for analysis.

<u>Soil</u> This test involves taking a soil sample to determine how much lead is in soil. It is sent to a lab for analysis.

<u>Water</u> This test determines how much lead is in water. The sample is sent to a lab for analysis.

Tests to Determine the Presence of Lead Paint.

<u>XRF</u> This test can only be done by a certified professional inspector using an XRF machine. It is like an x-ray machine that "reads" the amount of lead on a surface.

<u>Chip</u> This test takes a sample of paint down to the material on which it is applied. The chip then gets sent to a lab for analysis.

<u>Chemical</u> This test exposes paint to a chemical that turns color if lead is present.

Dust Wipe Sampling

Most children poisoned by lead paint are exposed because they get lead dust on their hands, toys, etc. and then put them in their mouths. Dust wipe sampling is an excellent way of determining if there is a lead hazard. Dust sampling will not tell you if there is lead paint on your walls and trim. Dust could come from outside.

The method described below is not as exact as the HUD protocol. **⑥** The purpose of this dust test is to locate a potential poisoning <u>before</u> it <u>happens</u>, and to test the effectiveness of a clean-up.

Any **pre-1978 house** that has a pregnant woman or a child under 6 years old either living there or frequently visiting, and has failing paint or was recently renovated, should be tested.

There are three other times you might take a dust test:

1. **Pre-Test**—before any work is done. This determines if there is a **dust hazard** and allows a comparison with levels after work is completed.
2. **Post Test**—after work and final clean-up. This test determines the levels of lead dust after work is complete. Unless you are doing the work yourself, it is best if this test is done as a "clearance test" by a professional "third party." This means the person who does the test is trained, in many states certified, and is unrelated to the person who did the work. "Third party" results carry more weight in a court of law. This test should be done according to HUD protocol. **⑥**
3. **A few months after work is completed to see if dust levels have gone back up**—You may want to monitor dust levels every year after that.

What rooms to sample:
- Where children spend the most time—the bedroom, kitchen, playroom, porch, etc.
- At the most-used entrance door.
- Where there are areas of failing paint.
- In an area where you have started or are planning to do work.

Spots in the room to sample:

- The window stool (the inside sill).
- The window trough—the part of the window sill between the window stool and the frame of the storm window, if there is a storm window.
- The floor—choose a spot out of most traffic, near a window. You can do this test on a carpet if there is no bare floor in a room.
- The floor in front of the most-used entrance.

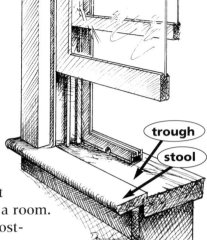

Materials you need:

- Baby or hand wipes—Use thin wipes that pull through a hole in the top of the container (avoid wipes with aloe, scent or alcohol).
- Zip lock freezer bags (about 4" x 5") OR a 35 mm film container or centrifuge tube. You can buy the tube from the lab you are using. (The film container or centrifuge tube will give you a more accurate reading, important when exact numbers are critical.)
- A permanent, fine-tip felt marking pen.
- Disposable gloves.
- A tape measure or ruler.
- A mailing envelope.
- Sample form—To record and identify the samples. The form is in Appendix **A**. Make copies.

How many samples to take and from where:

It is desirable to take separate samples from troughs, stools and floors in several rooms. For example: a trough, stool and floor in child's room, living room and kitchen. You can take one sample from each area of each room separately and send them to the lab, or you can take a "composite sample" (see p. 55).

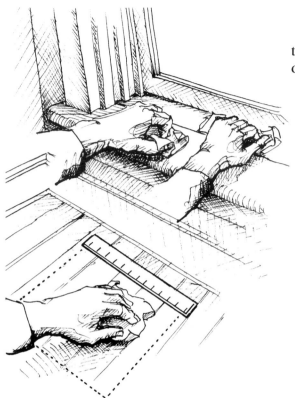

How to take a sample:

Throw away the first baby wipe that is sticking out because it may be dirty and dried out, then sample the . . .

Floor

1. Measure a 12" (12 inch) by 12" area. You may lay a ruler down along one side and use tape to mark off the exact area to be wiped.
2. Wipe the 12" square in one direction, side to side, in a zig-zag motion. (Try to wipe the entire surface with a minimum of overlap.) Use an even, moderate amount of pressure.
3. Fold the wipe, dirty side in, and wipe the same square in the same way in the opposite direction (top to bottom).
4. Place wipe in baggie, label baggie and enter information on form as described on the next page.

Stool

Same as floor except instead of a 12" by 12" square, wipe entire stool (in both directions), measure length and width, and enter dimensions on form.

Trough

Same as stool. If the window does not have a storm window, you can measure and wipe part of the sill.

Entrance sample:

To determine if lead dust is being tracked in, take a separate dust sample from the floor in front of the door most used. Do not composite this sample.

How to take a composite sample:

You can put up to four dust wipes in one container (be sure the lab you have chosen will take composite samples). All dust wipes put in the same container must be from the same building component. For example:

- You can put four wipes from four different floor areas in one container.
- You CAN NOT put a wipe from a floor and a wipe from a stool in the same container.
- Four is the maximum number of wipes you can put in a container.

ADVANTAGE: You save money because you pay the same for one wipe as for four wipes in a container.

DISADVANTAGE: One area could have high levels and another low. The composite method will only give you an average reading.

If you want specific information on any one spot, take a separate wipe from that spot and place it in a container by itself.

How to label the container and fill out form:

Copy the form from Appendix A to use for each house or apartment you test.

The address, number of sample and, if a composite sample is being collected, letter code for each location should appear on the label.

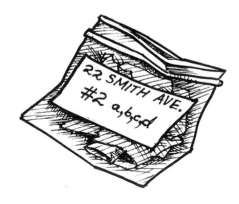

A

1, 2, and 3 are composite samples
5 through 8 are single samples

Check desired turn around time: 7 days____ 3 days ✔ 24 hours____

LAB: Please enter results in this column

SAMPLE NUMBER	IF COMPOSITE	NAME OF ROOM	BUILDING COMPONENT (floor, trough, stool, etc.)	DIMENSION OF SURFACE SAMPLED	SMOOTH	ROUGH	CARPET	LAB RESULT µg/ft'	ABOVE CLEARANCE
1	a	front bedroom	floor	12" x 12"			✔		
	b	rear "		" x "			✔		
	c	play room		" x "		✔			
	d	living room		" x "	✔				
2	a	front b.r.	stool	36" x 28"	✔				
	b	rear b.r.		34" x 28"	✔				
	c	play		4" x 30"		✔			
	d	living		4½" x 32"	✔				
3	a	front b.r.	trough	4" x 28"	✔				
	b	rear b.r.		4" x 28"	✔				
	c	play		4½" x 30"	✔				
	d	living		5" x 31"	✔				
4	a			" x "					
	b			" x "					
	c			" x "					
	d			" x "					
5		rear entrance	floor	12" x 12"	✔				
6		garage	floor	12" x 12"	✔				
7		basement	work bench	12" x 12"					
8		porch	deck	12"					
9									
10									

Round measurements off to nearest ½″

Where to mail samples:

Samples may be sent to any labs that:

- Are recognized by NLLAP (National Lead Laboratory Accreditation Program). A list of these labs can be obtained by calling 1-800-424-5323 (the National Lead Information Center Clearinghouse).
- Will take composite tests (up to four samples per container).
- Will accept samples in a baggie. Some labs will only accept samples in centrifuge tubes. They will supply you with the tubes.
- Charge less than $10 per individual or composite sample.

(See Appendix **F** for lab suggestions.)

What lab results mean:

The lab report will label samples in µg/ft². This stands for micrograms of lead in the dust wiped up from one square foot of surface. (If a sample is more or less than a square foot, the lab will do the calculations.)

Clearance levels:

HUD has set what it calls "clearance levels." These levels are considered the maximum acceptable levels after work has been done and the house has been professionally cleaned. A non-professional cleaning may not achieve these levels but should get as close as possible. Final payment on any lead or renovation work performed by a contractor should be based on achieving these levels:

below 100 μg/ft.² for floors
below 500 μg/ft.² for window stools
below 800 μg/ft.² for window troughs

Call your state information contact to check if local clearance levels are the same. **F**

We do not know exactly what a "safe level" is. Levels lower than these may be unhealthy, but levels greater than these, particularly on the floor where a child spends time, are certainly dangerous.

What to do about the results:

If there are high lead levels in the dust, and particularly if children are present, it is important to clean up the dust and address the causes of paint failure. This is usually a moisture problem. When possible, consult someone who has had formal training. At a minimum, all horizontal surfaces should be cleaned and, where possible, vacuumed with a HEPA vac. **①** See Appendix **B** for details.

Where further dust sampling reveals that levels are still high, the area should be recleaned and resampled. Remember, cleaning dust without addressing the cause of the dust will not solve the problem in the long run. It is critical to fix any peeling paint and address the causes before cleaning (see Chapter 2). Removing lead paint incorrectly can create more problems than it solves. The goal is to keep all paint intact and lead dust levels below clearance levels.

Again, "clearance levels" are to be achieved after work and special cleaning is done. Levels slightly above this may not be a health risk except where children are at an age where they spend time on the floor. Where levels above clearance are found it is particularly important to have a child's blood tested. Levels that are several times clearance levels are certainly a dangerous condition for children.

XRF Testing

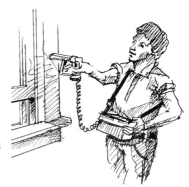

If your paint is in good condition, dust tests come back very low, and you do not plan to tear out painted surfaces, then there is probably no need to do an XRF test. If you are going to tear out some painted surfaces, you can assume they are lead or you can mail in a chip sample (see next page) rather than hiring a professional to do an XRF test.

The XRF test <u>must</u> be done by a trained and licensed professional. The tests are done as part of a formal lead inspection.

The inspector holds the XRF to a surface. The machine gives a reading. The reading is in mg/cm^2, which stands for milligrams of lead per square centimeter. The HUD standard is: anything at or over 1.0 mg/cm^2 or 0.5% by weight is considered lead paint. (This level may be lower in some states.)

The inspector can test each surface of a house or sample surfaces such as one wall, door, and window and the ceiling and floor (if painted) in each room. The test determines how much, if any, lead is present in all the paint layers. An XRF test may not be accurate. If any of the XRF readings are inconclusive, chip tests should be done.

What the results mean:

An XRF inspection report that reveals there is lead paint on specific surfaces does <u>not</u> necessarily mean that there is a risk.

There is a risk if the paint contains lead levels over the HUD standard <u>and</u> is chipping, flaking or being rubbed off. There will also be a risk if any architectural components are to be removed or demolished. Even the smallest amount of lead in paint will become extremely hazardous if it is burned or sanded.

The probability of architectural components having high lead levels is likely in the following order:

- exterior trim
- exterior siding
- bathroom and kitchen trim
- other interior trim
- bathroom and kitchen walls
- other walls and ceilings

most likely

to

least likely

> **Belt sanding or burning old paint with <u>any</u> level of lead content may create an extreme hazard.**

> **Remember, there can be lead paint present several layers down.**
> **If it is undisturbed and remains sealed, it does not represent a <u>risk.</u>**

Chip Testing

A chip test involves removing paint and sending it to a lab. The lab measures the percentage of lead in the sample. It is very accurate, but damages the surfaces you're testing. Taking many chip tests may also be expensive. Take a chip test if:

1. A surface is to be removed, scraped, sanded, or demolished, and you do not want to assume it's lead paint.
2. A surface is flaking or chipping and you want to know if it is lead paint. It is particularly important to test paint on old painted toys, cribs, etc.

When testing floors, the floor can be scraped and paint chips can be swept up with a small paint brush and put in a container.

Varnish or shellac may be too thin to get a chip for testing. You can sand a couple of inches and do a wipe test. This will only determine if there is lead present, not how much.

To take a chip test:

1. Measure an area about 2" by 2" on the wall or molding you want to test.

2. Tape baggie to the surface below the area to be sampled. Fold the part of the bag that is against the wall so the front of the bag stays open.

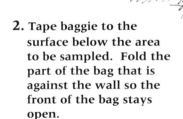

3. Cut, with sharp utility knife, the four edges down to the painted surface. It may be easier if you heat up (but not burn) the paint with a heat gun, or hair dryer, first. Avoid breathing any fumes.

4. With a sharp chisel remove all the paint, down to the unpainted surface, into the baggie. Scrape paint residue off with the back of the chisel.

5. Close up the baggie, label it with sample number and address, and enter info on sample form. **A**

Results—Anything over 0.5% or 500 µg/g (micrograms per gram), or 500 mg/kg (milligrams per kilogram) or 5,000 ppm (parts per million by weight), is considered to be lead paint. Lead paint may contain as much as 50% lead.

Peeling Paint - Remove pieces of the peeling paint and scrape the next layer down. This will indicate the amount of lead in the exposed and peeling paint. If the peeling paint or the layer directly below it is lead paint, particularly a paint with a high percentage of lead, there is a hazard. If this paint is not lead, there may still be lead in the paint several layers further down, but it is probably not a hazard. It may become a hazard, however, if the source of peeling is not repaired. (Just taking the top layers does not conform to the HUD-protocol chip test. **⑥**)

Always wet clean the area of the test when you have finished.

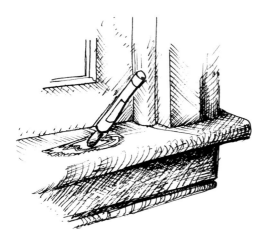

Chemical Testing

The purpose of this test is similar to the chip test. It is cheaper since you do not need to send a sample to the lab, and it can be purchased from a hardware store. But it only tells you if there is lead in the paint, not how much. Some tests may not be very accurate. It may tell you there is lead paint where there is none.

To use, follow the manufacturer's instructions exactly. For more information consult *Consumer Reports*, July, 1995.

Water Testing

Most houses, even older houses, do not have dangerous amounts of lead in the water. However, even new homes can have high levels of lead in water. Lead in water may come from:
- The municipal water supply
- The water pipes coming into your house
- The pipes and fixtures inside your house
- A well

You can call your municipal water department to find out the level of lead in the municipal water system. They may also know if your neighborhood tends to have lead pipes bringing water into houses.

Taking water samples is easy. Take samples from the tap most often used for drinking. Take one sample of water that has not been run for at least 6 hours. Take water from a cold water tap and make sure to get the first water out of the tap. To find out the lead content of water coming into the house, let it run for a few minutes, until water feels cold, then collect some in a different container.

Use a small plastic container with a screw-on lid, and put plastic wrap over the mouth of the jar before you put on the lid. This will prevent leaking. Send at least a cup of water to the lab.

What the results mean:

EPA's limit for lead in drinking water is 15 ppb (parts per billion) or 15 µg/L (micrograms per liter). The water department should be notified of levels above this.

If the first sample has high levels from plumbing in your house, let the water run for a few minutes before using (if it has not been used recently). If the second sample is high, notify your water department. Buy a water filter or bottled spring water for drinking, cooking, and particularly formula. Be aware that a water filter that is not correctly maintained will not be effective. Not all water filters remove lead. Only use water from the cold water tap for drinking and cooking.

Soil Testing

Most lead gets into soil from the normal chalking, peeling, and weathering of lead-based paint on a home or from industrial emissions. Sandblasting or burning off exterior leaded paint on buildings adds <u>dangerous</u> levels of lead to soil and air. Some lead contamination of soil remains from when there was lead in gasoline.

All soil contains some lead. Lead in soil does not move easily; it stays on the soil surface for years. Some of it runs off with topsoil during heavy rainstorms. Lead in soil is measured in parts per million (ppm).

The soil to be concerned about is bare soil, particularly bare soil where children play. Both direct contact and soil tracked into the house present a risk.

Where lead is found

The highest amount of lead in soil is usually found around homes painted with lead-based paint, near roadways, on sites of old factories or smelters that used lead in the past, and waste disposal areas. High levels are also found where old wood frame houses have been demolished. Soil near steel structures like bridges that have been sandblasted or have peeling painted surfaces is likely to be contaminated. Playgrounds near roadways or painted buildings may also contain lead.

If you are concerned about public play areas or school lots, request test sampling be paid for by the agency responsible for the area.

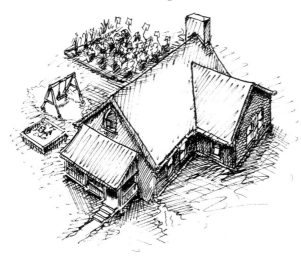

Where to test

The most important spots to sample are:

- Along the drip line (under roof edge) of a house, particularly at downspouts.
- Child's play areas, particularly where soil is bare.
- Gardens where food is grown.
- Near roadways.

Start by drawing a site plan of your home and choosing where you will take samples. Mark those spots on the plan. For example:

Composite samples (1A-1D) at the drip line
Garden samples (2)
Play area samples (3)
Sandbox sample (4)

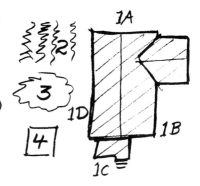

Testing and Sampling

Take two tablespoons of soil from an area measuring about 1 square inch. Put in a zip lock baggie. For composite sampling, take a sample from each chosen area (matched to the site plan) and put them in a zip lock baggie.

Label baggie with:
- Your address.
- Location of the sample or samples (matched to the plan).Then double-bag the samples for strength and mail to the lab. You can use the form in Appendix **A**.

Results

Soil test results are expressed in micrograms of lead per gram of soil ($\mu g/g$). This is equivalent to parts per million (ppm). Some laboratories may report concentrations as a percent of weight. This can be converted to $\mu g/g$ by moving the decimal point four places to the right:

.5% = 5,000 $\mu g/g$ = 5,000 ppm

No specific health standards exist yet, but in 1996 the EPA published "health based guidelines" for soil action levels:

400 ppm—where there is bare soil and frequent contact by children.
Action: Eliminate contact or cover with sod, grass, etc.

2,000 ppm—where there is bare residential soil but no contact by children.
Action: Cover with sod, grass, etc.

5,000 ppm—maximum level for bare residential soil.
Action: Abate the soil by removing the top few inches or permanently covering with concrete or asphalt.

Testing and Sampling Forms

COVER FORM SEND THIS COVER SHEET WITH ALL SAMPLE FORMS

MAKE COPIES OF THE FORMS YOU ARE GOING TO USE. ONE COPY OF THE COVER FORM BELOW SHOULD BE ATTACHED AND KEPT WITH THE FORMS YOU USE.

It is very important to fill out the form completely, legibly, and carefully. Results that are grossly inaccurate can either put children at risk or generate costly, unnecessary work.

Remember samples have two purposes: 1. to discover high risk situations and 2. give workers "as-is" and "post-work" comparative numbers. This allows them to evaluate the effectiveness of their work. A dust test done by an uncertified person may not qualify as a clearance test.

Street Address/Apt. Number: _____

City, State, Zip: _____

Owner Name: _____

Owner Phone Number:_____

Occupant Name: _____

Occupant Phone Number:_____

Are there children under seven years old present?_____

Is there peeling paint in the unit?_____

If yes, how much and where?_____

_____

_____

_____

_____

_____

Fax results to:_ _____

Mail results to: _____

_____

_____

_____

Check desired turn-around time: 7 days_____ 3 days_____ 24 hours _____

Collected by _____Date ____ / ____ /____
                         Signature

Mailed by _____Date ____ / ____ / ____
                         Signature

Results received by _____ Date ____ / ____ /____
                         Signature

This form may be copied without permission. Community Resources, Baltimore, Maryland

DUST SAMPLES

SAMPLE NUMBER	IF COMPOSITE	NAME OF ROOM	BUILDING COMPONENT (floor, trough, stool, etc.)	DIMENSIONS OF SURFACE SAMPLED	CONDITION SMOOTH	CONDITION ROUGH	CONDITION CARPET	LAB RESULT µg/ft²	ABOVE CLEARANCE
1	a b c d			" x " " x " " x " " x "					
2	a b c d			" x " " x " " x " " x "					
3	a b c d			" x " " x " " x " " x "					
4	a b c d			" x " " x " " x " " x "					
5				" x "					
6				" x "					
7				" x "					
8				" x "					
9				" x "					
10				" x "					
11				" x "					
12				" x "					

HUD Clearance Levels are: 100µg - Floors, 500µg - Stools, 800µg - Troughs

As is dust test ☐   Post work dust test ☐

This form may be copied without permission. Community Resources, Baltimore, Maryland

CHIP SAMPLES

SAMPLE NUMBER	LOCATION OF SAMPLE	SIZE	SURFACE SAMPLE	TO SUBSTRATE	PAINT CONDITION ✓							LAB RESULTS mg/cm² or %	ABOVE STANDARD
					SOUND	CRACKED	FLAKING	DELAMINATION	SUBSTRATE FAILURE	STRUCTURE FAILURE			
1													
2													
3													
4													
5													
6													

Paint is classified as lead paint if it is over 1.0 mg/cm² or 0.5% (also 5,000 ppm or 5,000 ug/g).

WATER SAMPLES

SAMPLE NUMBER	LOCATION OF FAUCET	FIRST DRAW SAMPLE (after not running water for 6 hours)	SECOND DRAW SAMPLE ✓	MUNICIPAL SUPPLY LEVEL (if known)	LAB RESULT ppb	ABOVE STANDARD ✓
1						
2						
3						

EPA action level is 15 PPB.

This form may be copied without permission. Community Resources, Baltimore, Maryland

SOIL SAMPLES

SAMPLE NUMBER	IF COMPOSITE	LOCATION (see plan)	CHILD'S AREA	NEXT TO HOUSE	DISTANCE FROM HOUSE (in feet)	BARE	COVERED	LAB RESULT ppm	ABOVE STANDARD
1	a				=				
	b				=				
	c				=				
	d				=				
2	a				=				
	b				=				
	c				=				
	d				=				
3	a				=				
	b				=				
	c				=				
	d				=				
4									
5									
6									

HUD Interim Standards: 400 for children's play area, 2,000 for building perimeter and yard. If over 5,000, cover or remove top layer.

Correct Cleaning
Appendix B

Cleaning Procedures

Renovation, painting or abatement work that breaks lead-painted surfaces and is done incorrectly can greatly increase lead poisoning risks for both workers and children returning to the home. Correct clean-up is crucial after any work on potentially lead-painted surfaces. The job is only as good as the final clean-up.

Frequency

This cleaning should always be done after work that breaks lead-painted surfaces. Decisions about whether or not, or how often this level of cleaning must be done, are best based on doing lead dust wipe tests to see if there is a presence or re-accumulation of lead dust.

The nature of lead dust

Lead dust is very fine and may be too fine to see. Where you can see paint chips, there is probably lead dust. But even if you cannot see chips, there may still be lead dust. A regular vacuum cleaner may pick up most of what a HEPA vac ① can pick up, but some of the finest dust will blow back out again. If large amounts of paint debris will be picked up, a HEPA vac is recommended. A HEPA vac is also recommended in homes where persons have respiratory problems.

Lead dust is sticky. You can't brush it off, it needs to be rubbed off. If rags, mop heads and rinse water are not changed often, the dust will just be smeared around rather than removed.

Lead dust accumulates in cracks over the life of a house. If these cracks are not cleaned out and sealed up, the dust filters back out of the cracks into the room after cleaning. Where there are wide spaces in tongue-and-groove flooring, each crack should be cleaned with a corner tool on a vacuum cleaner.

Equipment needed
- 4 cotton mop heads for each 2,000 sq. ft.
- 1 mop handle for mop head.
- 3 pails, one with mop squeezer (not a wringer bucket ⑦). See **F** for a less expensive squeeze bucket.
- 1 cleaning cloth per window plus 2 per room (a terry cloth towel cut into 10" x 10" squares works well).
- Cleaning detergent. There are lead-specific cleaners, designed to clean up lead dust **F**, but avoid TSP ⑧. If rinse water is changed frequently, a regular household cleaner works well.
- Vacuum or HEPA vac with floor brush, corner tool, and round cap brush.
- Tack cloths for finished furniture. These can be purchased in hardware stores.
- Paper towels.
- Latex gloves.
- Small plastic jug (1 quart) or small spray bottle.

Correct Cleaning

The Clean-up
It's important that things are done in this order and no steps are left out:

1) **Children**
   All children should be out of the house or apartment during cleaning.

2) **Rugs**
   Remove rugs and send to be cleaned. Wear at least a NIOSH-approved mask (p. 40) when rolling up rugs. HEPA vac or vacuum the area under each rug as soon as it is removed. Misting rugs before rolling them up keeps down dust. Rolling the rugs in plastic prevents the spreading of dust.

3) **Wall-to-wall carpets**
   Wall-to-wall carpeting cannot be well cleaned. It tends to contain mold, mildew, and dust mites. It can gather food particles which attract roaches. It can also gather lead dust. Unless it is kept dry, cleaned often with a good vacuum cleaner and replaced as necessary, it can become a health hazard ③.

   It is recommended that wall-to-wall carpet that is not fairly new be disposed of and replaced with area rugs for rooms and runners for halls and staircases. The more bare floor is accesable and sealed the easier it is to clean.

   To dispose of wall-to-wall carpet, you must wear at least a NIOSH-approved mask. Close doors to the rest of the house and seal them with tape before you start. Cleaning equipment should be in the room before it is sealed. Clean up before unsealing and opening door. Carpet carried out through the house should be wrapped in poly first. Any furniture that must be left should be covered with poly and well cleaned after removing carpet. This is particularly important for upholstered furniture. If you keep wall-to-wall carpets, the companies with truck-mounted vacuum machines will do the best job of cleaning. If you wet-clean carpets, use fans, heat and open windows to speed up drying time to prevent mold growth.

4) **Cloth**
   Remove all contaminated cloth (curtains, spreads, child's blanket, clothing on the floor, etc.) and send to be cleaned.

5) **Objects in room**
   Prepare a small bucket of mild cleaner or use tack cloth to wipe down as many small objects on shelves, bureaus, window stools, etc. as possible and put into boxes. You can leave things in dresser drawers, cabinets and closets if the paint in these spaces is in good condition.
   CAUTION: Water and detergent can mar furniture finish. Use tack cloths on finished furniture. These can be bought in a hardware store.

Correct Cleaning

6) Surfaces

HEPA vac or vacuum the unit from one end to the other, starting at the end farthest from the front door. Within each room start vacuuming from the top shelves, tops of doors, window casing, and other trim, then do every inch of the windows, particularly the trough. (Clean out trough with damp paper towels first to pick up paint chips and large pieces before vacuuming.) Vacuum upholstered furniture with a HEPA vac, including hard-to-reach crevices and under seat cushions. Then vacuum the floor using the corner tool where the floor meets the baseboard. Cracks between the floor boards should be cleaned with a corner tool. Use the round cup brush for all small surfaces. In most cases only horizontal surfaces need washing. The exception is in rooms where large amounts of lead dust have been generated, as in demolition, or where the wall surface is rough enough to hold dust.

7) Clean trim, windows and doors

- Pour cleaning solution (mix according to instructions) into a plastic jug or small sprayer.
- Dampen cloth squares by pouring the solution from the jug or misting the surface. (This avoids contaminating the cleaning solution.)
- Using two small buckets (one empty and one with rinse water), rinse out rag in bucket with rinse water, then squeeze dirty water into empty bucket.
- Change rinse water often. Throw away rag (or put in bag to be laundered) at least once in every room.
- Start from highest points and work down, cleaning windows, shelves, edges, mantels, top of moldings, etc. in each room.
- When cleaning windows, wash trough with paper towels first.
  Never use the rag you used on a window for other areas because you may spread dust.

8) Floors—The sequence is:

1. Mist floor with detergent from pump spray container or dip mop head in detergent bucket, then ring out. Keep detergent water as clean as possible.
2. Wash floor. If floor is very dirty, scrub with mop, then rinse mop in rinse bucket. Squeeze out excess water into squeezer or twist bucket. If you are using twist mop, squeeze into empty bucket. **Never put mop into the dirty water that was squeezed out of the mop.** Rinse and squeeze again. Change rinse water often.
3. Again spray detergent on floor or dip mop in detergent water, then clean, rinse, squeeze, etc.
4. For rinsing floor, clean out buckets and repeat washing procedures but replace detergent with clean water. Do three to five rooms with one mop head, then throw it away or wash it. Use new mop head on those same rooms for rinsing.

FOR SMALL JOBS OR WEEKLY CLEANING

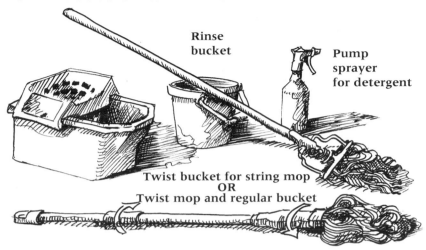

Rinse bucket

Pump sprayer for detergent

Twist bucket for string mop
OR
Twist mop and regular bucket

FOR LARGE JOBS

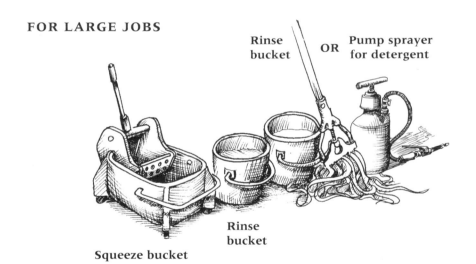

Rinse bucket

OR Pump sprayer for detergent

Rinse bucket

Squeeze bucket

9) Weekly cleaning

Maintain house by weekly cleaning, particularly the window troughs. When cleaning window troughs, use damp paper towels to pick up visible dirt, then follow with rags. Do not use these rags on other surfaces. Thoroughly clean stools and around baseboards. If there is any peeling or flaking paint, it should be dealt with (see wet scraping instructions on p. 25); meanwhile, at least keep any loose chips cleaned up. Damp mop all rooms, changing mop heads every few months. As much as possible, keep all surfaces smooth and cleanable.

Safely isolating the work area until after final clean-up is crucial for both do-it-yourselfers and professionals.

Some of the most severe poisonings of children have been due to their being home during or following a renovation or paint job. Even an "abated house" improperly isolated and cleaned can present a greater hazard than doing nothing. (One documented "abatement" that was not cleaned up properly increased dust levels from 20µg/sq. ft. to 2000 µg/sq. ft., a 100-fold increase.)

A reminder about prohibited work practices: dry scraping, burning, sanding (particularly power sanding), water blasting, unprotected chemical stripping and uncontained demolition are particularly hazardous.

There is no way to be sure how much dust a particular work practice will create without hiring a professional to measure the airborne dust during work ⑤. Therefore the following is only a suggestion of possible risk.

Risk is divided into three categories. It is recommended that the high-risk work be done by a person who has attended at least a two-day EPA workers training course and is supervised by a person who has attended the EPA four-day supervisor training. For more about site protection, particularly low and moderate-risk work, see Chapter 5. For more detail read the HUD guidelines. **F**

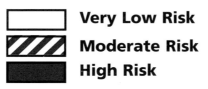

Very Low Risk

Moderate Risk

High Risk

For low-risk measures, all that is needed is to put plastic below work area extending five feet in each direction. Before you move plastic from one room to another:

- Pick up large scraps with damp paper towels or mist then gently sweep up.
- Vacuum up fine dust with the brush attachment. Use a HEPA vac if available.
- Carefully fold up plastic, dirty side in, then move to next work area.

Keep doors and windows closed, if possible, to keep paint chips from blowing off plastic. Wear booties, to be removed when stepping off plastic, or remove shoes to avoid tracking chips and dust. Clean up immediately following work.

Site Protection

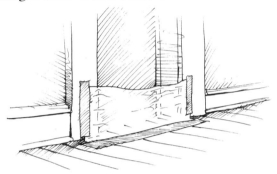 Any dust or chips created by moderate-level work, like wet scraping paint from an entire room, should be confined to that room. Any furniture left in the room should be covered. If the floor has cracks or may be hard to clean, it should be covered with 6 mil polyethylene sheeting which is taped to the baseboard.

To keep dust from traveling to other rooms, the doors should be kept closed, especially if there is a window open, since opening a door could blow dust into the rest of the house.

When small amounts of dust are being generated, tape plastic across bottom of door. Remove shoes or shoe covers (booties), when leaving the room.

The most effective way to contain dust within a room while still allowing access, is to construct a double-layer door cover, as illustrated.

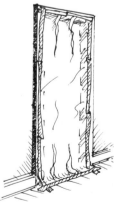 **1.** Using duct tape, tape 6 mil plastic to perimeter of door. Leave the plastic a couple of inches long so it can be easily taped to the floor. Leave about a foot of slack in plastic so it is not pulled tight over opening. You may staple corners to molding for strength.

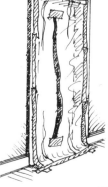 **2.** Make a slice in the plastic starting about 6" from the top of the door jamb and ending about 6" from the floor. Run a short piece of duct tape across the top and bottom of cut to prevent the plastic from ripping.

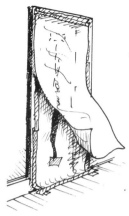

3. Tape, and staple at corners, a second layer of plastic to the top of the door jamb. Cut it about an inch short of the floor so it lays against the first sheet of plastic.

Before stepping through the opening, remove booties or shoes and take off Tyvek® suit or vacuum off clothes. In all cases, the room in which work is being done should be vacuumed at the end of each day. The entire house should be fully cleaned at the end of the job.

It is critical whenever dust is created that the vents in a forced air system, particularly the return vent, be sealed with plastic and duct tape.

▮▮▮▮ High levels of dust created by demolition or use of power tools need to be completely isolated from living spaces. This means that there should be no direct passage between the work area and the living space before the work area is completely cleaned and dust tests indicate clearance levels have been achieved.

If any furniture is left in the work space it must be covered with plastic, which is then taped to the floor with duct tape.

The work space should be shut off from living spaces by closing a door, locking it and taping the perimeter with duct tape. If there is no door, use a sheet of plywood. Workers enter and exit the space through a different door. If the room on the first, second or third floor, a ladder may be used for access.

If this is not possible, construct two double-layer door covers on both ends of a space just outside the work space (see above). Workers would leave the area through this small space, remove Tyvek® suits, vacuum themselves and/or change clothes and clean up. At least wash pails would be placed in this area so workers could clean up before going through the second barrier, into the living space.

At the end of the job, the work area and then the rest of the house should be cleaned up **B** then dust tested. Children should not enter these work areas until successful clearance dust test results are returned from the lab.

Appendix D

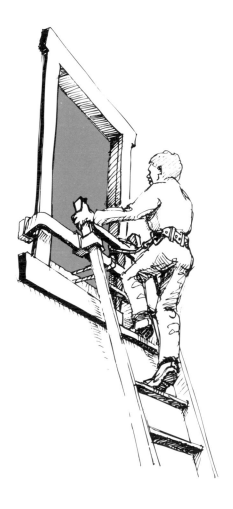

LADDER SAFETY

Before using a ladder, be sure the ladder has rubber feet and is in good condition.

- To work on windows, attach a "stand off" to top of ladder. It will span window and bear on wall on both sides of window. This puts the worker in the center of window leaning in, not out.
- Cut through poly drop cloth and place the rubber feet of ladder directly on ground, never on poly.
- When raising a tall ladder it is good to have someone helping from the window with a rope tied to top of ladder.
- To secure ladder, tie rung at sill height to a 2x4 on the inside stool that extends well past casing on both sides. Pull rope tight and tie off.
- Workers should tie themselves off to a rung above them with the lanyard (rope) of a safety belt. Leave minimum of slack in lanyard.
- Before using ladder, check feet, rungs and frame.

EYES

Always wear goggles when you are:
- scraping
- cutting with power tools
- using strippers
- doing demolition
- working overhead
- using case-hardened nails

All worksites should have a place to wash out eyes.

HEAT

Working indoors in hot weather can be very hot, particularly when the work area is closed up and workers are wearing respirators and protective suits. It is important to guard against heat stroke and heat stress. Heat stroke is a medical emergency.

HEAT STROKE

Danger signs to look for:
- Hot, dry skin, sweating stops, suit dries
- Fainting
- Headache/dizziness
- Sick to stomach

Action to take:
- Call for ambulance and tell them it is a heat stroke emergency.
- Remove individual from work area.
- Remove respirator/suit.
- Cool body with water or ice.

HEAT STRESS

Danger signs to look for:
- Cool, sweaty, pale skin
- Headache, dizziness, sick to stomach

Action to take:
- Remove individual from work area.
- If fainting, call ambulance.
- Remove respirator/suit.
- Do not give water to a person who has fainted.
- Cool body with water.

PREVENTING THE PROBLEM

- Drink lots of water
- Get used to heat gradually
- Drink orange juice and eat bananas before work and during breaks
- Cut down on alcohol
- Take breaks
- Maintain a flow of air through the worksite, but make sure lead dust does not contaminate other areas.

Essential maintenance practices for property owners and standard treatments as outlined in the Title X Task Force report ▣ may not be sufficient to maintain a lead-safe house, but they are useful as minimum requirements. You may use them as a checklist for evaluating a property owner's work practices.

ESSENTIAL MAINTENANCE PRACTICES FOR PROPERTY OWNERS

1. Use safe work practices during work that may contain lead to avoid creating LBP hazards.
- Do not use unsafe paint removal practices, including:
  - Open flame burning;
  - Power sanding or sandblasting (unless a special vacuum attachment is used to contain dust);
  - Water blasting; and
  - Dry scraping more than a minor surface area (for example, more than one square foot per room).
- Use good work practices and take precautions to prevent the spread of lead dust (for example, limit access to the work area only to workers; cover the work area with six millimeter polyethylene plastic or equivalent; protect workers; protect occupant's belongings by covering or removing from the work area; wet painted surfaces before disturbing; and wet debris before sweeping).
- Perform specialized cleaning of the work area upon completion of work using methods designed to remove lead-contaminated dust.

2. Perform visual examinations for deteriorating paint (unless the paint is found not to be LBP).
- At unit turnover; and
- Every 12 months (unless the tenant refuses entry).

3. Promptly and safely repair deteriorated paint and the cause of the deterioration. If more than a minor amount of paint (for example, more than one square foot per room) has deteriorated (unless the paint is found not to be LBP):
- Make the surface intact by paint stabilization, enclosure, encapsulation, or removal.

- Follow Essential Maintenance Practice #1 (above) when repairing the surface.
- Diagnose and correct any physical conditions causing the paint deterioration (for example, structural and moisture problems causing substrate failure or conditions causing painted surfaces to be crushed).
- When there is extensive paint deterioration (for example, more than five square feet per room), the procedures for dust testing after Standard Treatments apply.

4. Provide generic LBP hazard information to tenants per Title X including the EPA-developed educational pamphlet and any information available about LBP or LBP hazards specific to the unit.

5. Post written notice to tenants asking tenants to report deteriorating paint and informing them whom to contact. Promptly respond to tenants' reports and correct deteriorating paint, with accelerated response in units occupied by a child under age six or a pregnant woman—and in no case longer than 30 days. Do not retaliate against tenants who report deteriorating paint.

6. Train maintenance staff. At a minimum, maintenance supervisors need to complete a one-day training course based on the HUD/EPA operations and maintenance/interim control activities curriculum. The maintenance supervisor must ensure that workers either take the one-day training course or have a clear understanding of LBP hazards, unsafe practices, occupant protection, and dust clean-up methods by such means as on-the-job training and video instruction. The maintenance supervisor needs to provide adequate oversight of workers who have not taken the training course.

STANDARD TREATMENT

1. Safely repair deteriorated paint. (Note that the safe repair of deteriorating paint should have already been done under Essential Maintenance Practices. The same procedures apply to stabilizing deteriorated paint identified in the course of Standard Treatments.)

2. Provide smooth and cleanable horizontal surfaces. Rough, pitted, and porous surfaces trap lead dust and make it difficult to thoroughly clean these surfaces. Smooth horizontal surfaces will make it possible for tenants' regular housekeeping to reduce exposure to lead dust (for example, recoating hardwood floors with polyurethane, replacing or recovering worn out linoleum floors, treating interior window sills). During treatment of an occupied unit, occupants and their possessions must be protected from lead exposure, but only surfaces that are accessible need to be treated.

3. Correct conditions in which painted surfaces are rubbing, binding, or being crushed that can produce lead dust (unless the paint is found not to be LBP). Owners shall correct conditions that cause rubbing, binding, or crushing of painted surfaces to protect the integrity of the paint and reduce the generation of lead dust (for example, rehanging binding doors, installing door stops to prevent doors from damaging painted surfaces, reworking windows).

4. Cover or restrict access to bare residential soil (unless it is found not to be lead-contaminated). Under Title X, only bare soil that is lead-contaminated is defined as a hazard. Owners shall visually check for bare soil when performing treatments on a unit and implement controls to prevent occupant exposure (for example, covering bare soil with gravel, mulch, or sod; physically restricting access to bare soil). In most cases, covering bare soil is an effective control.

5. Specialized cleaning. Lead-contaminated dust, the foremost path of childhood poisonings, may not be visible to the naked eye and is difficult to clean up. Owners shall conduct specialized cleaning of work areas upon completion of the treatments above. During treatment of an occupied unit, only surfaces that are accessible need to be cleaned.

6. Perform sufficient dust tests to ensure safety. When performing Standard Treatment in vacant units, sufficient dust tests are needed following treatment to provide a reasonable assurance of compliance. Dust tests of the work area are to be performed after completion of Standard Treatments in any unit occupied by a family with a child under age six or a pregnant woman if more than a de minimus amount of paint is disturbed.

The text shown above is drawn from the Title X Task Force Summary Report. The entire Summary can be purchased for $5.00 from HUD User at 800-245-2691. Ask for report HUD-1542-LBP, June 1995, or by title, Putting The Pieces Together - Summary.

Appendix F

Information Resource List

ALLIANCE TO END CHILDHOOD LEAD POISONING
227 Massachusetts Avenue NE, Suite 200
Washington, DC 20002
(202) 543-1147
Areas of expertise: The Alliance to End Childhood Lead Poisoning provides information on current and pending federal legislation and regulations. In addition, they distribute a number of publications on prevention issues.

NATIONAL LEAD INFORMATION CENTER (NLIC)
1025 Connecticut Avenue NW Suite 1200
Washington, DC 20036-5405
(800) 424-5323l
http://www.nsc.org/ehc/lead.htm
NLIC operates a toll-free lead hotline where information specialists respond to questions and provide more than 150 different documents to the public free of charge. The NLIC website includes an interactive document order form, a Spanish language page, current information on lead-related issues, past issues of the Lead Inform newsletter, and links to the best sources of lead information on the Internet.

HUD LEAD LISTING
The US Department of Housing and Urban Development has created the National Lead Service Providers Listing System to provide consumers with the means to identify and locate lead inspectors and risk assessors nationwide. For more information call, toll-free (888) LEAD-LIST or check their website at: http://www.leadlisting.org. You can also visit HUD's lead-based paint homepage at www.HUD,GOV/LEA for additional information.

NATIONAL CENTER FOR LEAD-SAFE HOUSING
10227 Wincopin Circle, Suite 205
Columbia, MD 21044
(410) 992-0712
Areas of expertise: Technical standards and assistance to local government lead poisoning prevention programs, and the real estate, finance, and insurance industries.

PARENTS AGAINST LEAD (PAL)
1438 E. 52nd Street
Chicago, IL 60615-4122
(773) 324-7824
An organization of and for parents of lead-poisoned children.

CONSERVATION LAW FOUNDATION
62 Summer Street
Boston, MA 02110
(617) 350-0990
Areas of expertise: State lead law database and technical assistance.

Select Product List

Product availability and prices may change. Call to confirm information.

GLIDWALL/INSUL AID
Mesh system for interior walls
Source: any local Glidden Paint Co.

GRIPPER PRIMER
A high adhesion primer for interior and exterior
Source: any local Glidden Paint Co.

GLOBAL ENCASEMENT
An encapsulation system for interior and exterior (includes primer, top coat and caulk). Applicator needs company certification for large jobs. Top coat can be used without primer for interior surfaces in moderate condition.
Source: Global Encasement (800) 230-7296

LEDIZOLV DETERGENT
Lead specific cleaner (alternative to TSP)
Source: Hin-Core Industries (704) 587 0744

LABS FOR LEAD SAMPLES
Both of the following labs are certified by the American Industrial Hygiene Association and the National Voluntary Laboratory Accreditation Program. In addition, both are participants in the Environmental Lead Proficiency Analytical Testing Program. For the names of other certified labs, call (800) 356-4674.

Source: ENVIRONMENTAL SERVICES Call (800) 347-4010, or check their website at http//www.enrlab.com. Will analyze chip, dust, or soil for $5, single or composite in baggies or tubes. 48-hour turnaround. .

Source: METS LABORATORIES (800) 604-1995 or visit their web site at metslaboratories.com
The METS Docuclean dust testing system is an easy to use pre-packaged kit consisting of tubes, wipes, return envelope, etc. for the collection of 5 single or 5 composite dust, paint chips or soil samples. Kits can be purchased for $4.00 each plus local tax. The analysis cost is $4.50 for each sample sent to the laboratory. METS offers a 24 hour turnaround time. Docuclean kits can be customized to include up to 100 samples to accomodate any size job.

JAMB LINERS 38" 54" 70" 80" *Vinyl compression track for sash (can be cut for single sash). Case of 25 @ $6.75 for 54"*
Source: J.R. Products (800) 343-4446

HEPA VAC
HEPA vacs, Euroclean UZ930 or UZ964H that you wear on your hip for approx..$340. Light HEPA Vac with 3 bag system Approx. $500. If you speak directly to Elaine Wax at extension 234, mention D. Livingston to her. Aramsco also makes quantity sales of shoe covers, tyvek® suits, dust masks, Ledizolv small mist bottles, 6 mil poly, etc.
Source: Aramsco (800) 767-6933

CHEMICAL TEST - LEADCHECK SWABS
Test for lead in paint, dust, tubs, blinds, dishes. (Ask for copy of "screening dust for clearance protocol")
Source: Hybrivet Systems Inc. (800) 262-5323

MOP BUCKET
Rhino Bucket with ringer, 15 quart. Product # 80 for $9.95 each, minimum order isone case of six.
Source: American Institutional Supplies (800) 866-3331

Please note: Mention of a product does not constitute endorsement by the author. The author has used these products and has been satisfied with their performance.

Recommended Documents

GETTING THE LEAD OUT
Irene Kessel, John T. O'Connor- Plenum
To order, call (800)221-9369 ext. 349, $18.95
A comprehensive book on the legal and medical aspects of lead poisoning. The book contains a state-by-state and topic-by-topic list of information sources.

PUTTING THE PIECES TOGETHER; CONTROLLING LEAD HAZARDS IN THE NATION'S HOUSING, THE SUMMARY
Lead-Based Paint Hazard Reduction and Financing Task Force
To order, call (800) 424-5323, Free
The most important document on national lead policy. Focusing on principles and specific recommendations.

GUIDELINES FOR THE EVALUATION AND CONTROL OF LEAD-BASED PAINT HAZARDS IN HOUSING
U.S. Department of Housing and Urban Development
To order, call (800) 245-2691, $45.00
To order select chapters call (800) 424-5323, Free
This is the comprehensive technical document on lead hazard remediation.

GUIDE TO INNOVATIVE FINANCING FOR CONTROL OF LEAD HAZARDS
Alliance to End Childhood Lead Poisoning
To order, call (202) 543-1147, $25.00 (Free to non-profits)
How to take advantage of the Community Reinvestment Act
A reference book for community organizations and policy development.

CREATING A LEAD-BASED PAINT HAZARD CONTROL POLICY
The National Center for Lead Safe Housing
To order, call Evelyne Bloomer at (410) 992-07112, $5.00
A practical step-by-step approach for non-profit housing organizations.

MASTERING THE BUSINESS OF REMODELING
Linda W. Case, Victoria L. Downing
To order, call, (301) 587-6343
An action plan for profit, progress, and peace of mind.

RESOURCE HANDBOOK ON LEAD HAZARD DISCLOSURE FOR HOMES AND APARTMENTS
Alliance to End Childhood Lead Poisoning
To order, call (202) 543-1147, $60.00
Step-by-step summary of disclosure process and practical advice for real estate agents, buyers, sellers, tenants, contractors and inspectors.

Recommended Documents

CHILDHOOD LEAD POISONING—BLUEPRINT FOR PREVENTION
Alliance to End Childhood Lead Poisoning
To order, call (202) 543-1147, $4.00
A overview of national and local strategies and policy recommendations.

THE HEALTHY HOME HANDBOOK
John Warde, Time Books, ISBN 0-8129-2151-8
To order, call (800) 733-3000, $17.00
A comprehensive and readable book on controlling indoor pollutants and minimizing safety hazards in the home.

IS THIS YOUR CHILD'S WORLD?
Dories J. Rapp MD, Bantam
To order, call (800) 323-9872, $24.95
How you can fix the schools and homes that are making your children sick. Help for children who are hyperactive, asthmatic, disruptive, or suffering from chronic colds or learning problems.

RUNNING A SUCCESSFUL CONSTRUCTION COMPANY
David Gerstel, Taunton Press
To order, call (203) 426-8171, $27.95
An extraordinarily good book for contractors and people who work with contractors.

HOME TECH REMODELING AND RENOVATION COST ESTIMATOR
Henry Reynolds, Home Tech
To order, call (800) 638-8292, $69.50 plus $4.50 shipping
The best guide for pricing renovation jobs.

PROFESSIONAL REMODELING MANAGEMENT
Walter Stoeppelwerth, Home Tech
To order, call (800) 638-8292, $37.50
A comprehensive book on contractor business management.

BUILDERS GUIDE
Joseph Lstiburek, Building Science Corporation
To order, call (978) 589-5100, $43.00 (includes shipping)
One book for each of four North American and Mexican climates: Cold, Mixed, Hot-humid, Hot-dry. The best books on the house as a system, dealing with moisure problems in new construction and construction principles.

SIMPLE STEPS TO A LEADSMART™ HOME VIDEO
LEQADSMART™ HOMES MULTIMEDIA CD-ROM
LEADSMART™ APARTMENT LEASING VIDEO
To order, call toll free (888) 532-3762, or check their website at
www.leadsmarthomes.com, $19.95-$39.95
If you are buying, selling or renovating a pre-1978 home, these user-friendly products will help you to protect your family's health and the economic investment in your home.

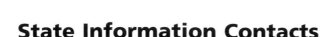

Resources

State Information Contacts

ALASKA
Dept of Health & Social
Services
PO Box 240249
3601 C St Ste 540
Anchorage AK 99524-0249
(907) 269-8044
Fax: (907) 562-7802

ALABAMA
Bureau of Environmental
Health
Dept of Public Health
434 Monroe St
Montgomery AL 36117
(334) 613-5200
Fax: (334) 240-3387

ARKANSAS
AR Dept of Health
Div of Environmental Health
4815 W Markham St Slot 46
Little Rock AR 72205-3867
(501) 661-2171
Fax: (501) 661-2572

ARIZONA
Bureau of Epidemiology &
Disease Control Services
3815 N Black Canyon Hwy
Phoenix AZ 85015
(602) 230-5808
Fax: (602) 230-5959

CALIFORNIA
Dept of Health Services
Childhood Lead Poisoning
5801 Christie Ave Ste 600
Emeryville CA 94608
(510) 450-2448
Fax: (510) 450-2442

COLORADO
CO Dept of Public Health
4300 Cherry Creek Dr S
Denver CO 80222-1530
(303) 692-2685
Fax: (303) 782-4969

CONNECTICUT
Dept of Public Health, Division
of Environmental Health

CONNECTICUT CONTD.
450 Capitol Ave
PO Box 340308 MS SI LED
Hartford CT 06134-0308
(860) 509-7293
Fax: (860) 509-7295

DISTRICT OF COLUMBIA
Environmental Regulation
2100 Martin Luther King Jr
Ste 203
Washington DC 20020
(202) 645-6617
Fax: (202) 645-6622

DELAWARE
Division of Public Health
Jesse S Cooper Bldg PO Box
Dover DE 19903
(302) 739-3028
Fax: (302) 739-3839

FLORIDA
Dept of Health
1317 Winewood Blvd
Tallahassee FL 32399-0700
(904) 487-2945
Fax: (904) 487-3729

GEORGIA
Dept of Human Resources
Environmental Health Section
2 Peachtree St 5th Fl Annex
Atlanta GA 30303-3186
(404) 657-6511
Fax: (404) 657-6533

HAWAII
Dept of Environmental Health
PO Box 3378
Honolulu HI 96801
(808) 586-4425
Fax: (808) 586-4444

IOWA
Dept of Public Health/Env
Childhood Lead Poisoning
Lucas State Office Bldg 1st
321 E 12th St
Des Moines IA 50319-0075
(515) 242-6340
Fax: (515) 281-4958

IDAHO
ID Dept of Environmental
Health
Towers Bldg 4th Fl PO Box
Boise ID 83720-0036
(208) 334-0606
Fax: (208) 334-6581

ILLINOIS
Dept of Public Health
Environmental Health
525 W Jefferson St
Springfield IL 62761
(217) 546-1896

INDIANA
Maternal & Child Health
Childhood Lead Poisoning
2 N Meridian
Indianapolis IN 46204
(317) 233-1232

KANSAS
Dept of Health & Environment
Bldg 283 Forbes Field
Topeka KS 66620-0001
(913) 296-1542
Fax: (913) 296-1545

KENTUCKY
Health Program Coordinator
Dept of Public Health
Div of Env Health &
275 E Main St
Frankfort KY 40621
(502) 564-4856
Fax: (502) 564-6533

LOUISIANA
LA Dept of Environmental
Health
5222 Summa Court
Baton Rouge LA 70809
(504) 765-2554
Fax: (504) 765-2559

MASSACHUSETTS
MA Dept of Public Health
Childhood Lead Poison
470 Atlantic Ave 2nd Fl
Boston MA 02210-2224

Resources

F

MASSACHUSETTS CONTD.
(617) 753-8401
Fax: (617) 753-8436

MARYLAND
MD Dept of the
Environment
2500 Broening Hwy Rm
2134
Baltimore MD 21224
(410) 631-3820
Fax: (410) 631-4186

MAINE
Bureau of Health
151 Capitol St State House
Augusta ME 04333
(207) 287-3290
Fax: (207) 287-4631

MICHIGAN
Public Health Agency
Dept of Community Health
3423 N Martin Luther King
Jr
PO Box 30195
Lansing MI 48909
(517) 335-8024
Fax: (517) 335-9476

MINNESOTA
MN Department of Health
717 Delaware St SE
Minneapolis MN 55414
(612) 215-0731
Fax: (612) 627-5479

MISSOURI
Dept of Health
Div Environmental
PO Box 570/930 Wildwood
Jefferson City MO
(573) 751-6102
Fax: (573) 526-6946

MISSISSIPPI
MS Dept of Env Quality
Air Division
PO Box 10385
Jackson MS 39289-0385
(601) 961-5164
Fax: (601) 961-5742

MONTANA
Planning/Prevention
Dept of Health and Env
1520 E 6th Ave
 Helena MT 59620-0901
(406) 444-5267
Fax: (406) 444-1374

NORTH CAROLINA
Dept of Health & Human
Services
PO Box 29601
Raleigh NC 27626
(919) 733-0820
Fax: (919) 733-8493

NORTH DAKOTA
Dept of Health
Environmental Health
Section
1200 Missouri Ave PO Box
Bismarck ND 58506-5520
(701) 328-5150
Fax: (701) 328-5200

NEBRASKA
NE Department of Health
HHS Regulation and
Licensure
301 Centennial Mass S.
PO Box 95007
Lincoln NE 68509-5007
(402) 471-0782
Fax: (402) 471-6436

NEW HAMPSHIRE
Division of Public Health
Childhood Lead Poison
6 Hazen Dr
Concord NH 03301-6501
(603) 271-4507
Fax: (603) 271-3745

NEW JERSEY
Environmental Health
3635 Quaker Bridge Rd
PO Box 369
Trenton NJ 08625-0369
(609) 588-3120
Fax: (609) 584-5370

NEW MEXICO
Lead Program
Dept of Health
1435 St Francis Dr
Santa Fe NM 87505
(505) 827-3709
Fax: (505) 827-3714

NEVADA
Dept of Health
Division of Epidemiology
505 E King St Rm 201
Carson City NV 89710
(702) 687-3786
Fax: (702) 687-3859

NEW YORK
NY Dept of Health
Bureau of Occupational
Health
1215 Western Ave Rm 205
Albany NY 12203-3399
(518) 458-6483
Fax: (518) 458-6469

OHIO
Lead Poisoning Prevention
Environmental Health
246 N High St
Columbus OH 43266-0588
(614) 644-8649
Fax: (614) 752-4157

OKLAHOMA
OK Dept of Environmental
Health
4545 N Lincoln Blvd Ste
250
Oklahoma City OK 73105-
3483
(405) 271-5220
Fax: (405) 962-2200

OREGON
Lead Program
800 NE Oregon St Ste 608
Portland OR 97262
(503) 731-4012
Fax: (503) 731-4077

PENNSYLVANIA
Dept of Health

State Information Contacts

PENNSYLVANIA CONTD.
Childhood Lead Poison
PO Box 90 Rm 725
Harrisburg PA 17108
(717) 783-8451
Fax: (717) 772-0323

PUERTO RICO
Emergency Response &
Environmental Quality Board
PO Box 11488
Santurce PR 00910
(809) 766-2823

RHODE ISLAND
Off of Env Health Risk
Assessment
RI Dept. of Env. Health
3 Capitol Hill Rm 208
Providence, RI 02908-5097
(401) 277-1417

SOUTH CAROLINA
Dept of Health
2600 Bull St
Columbia SC 29201
(803) 935-7894 Fax: (803)
935-7825

SOUTH DAKOTA
Dept of Env and Natural
Office of Waste Management
Joe Foss Bldg 523 E Capital
Pierre SD 57501-3181
(605) 773-3153
Fax: (605) 773-5286

TENNESSEE
Dept of Environment
Life and Casualty Tower
401 Church St 21st Fl
Nashville TN 37243-0435
(615) 532-0109
Fax: (615) 532-0120

TEXAS
Env Lead Branch
TX Dept of Health
Toxic Substances Control
1100 W 49th St
Austin TX 78756-3194

TEXAS CONTD.
(512) 834-6612
Fax: (512) 834-6644

UTAH
Division of Air Quality
Dept of Environmental
150 N 1950 W PO Box 144820
Salt Lake City UT
(801) 536-4085
Fax: (801) 536-4099

VIRGINIA
Childhood Lead Poison
1500 E Main St Rm 138
Richmond VA 23218-2448
(804) 225-4455
Fax: (804) 371-6031

VIRGIN ISLANDS
Dept of Planning and Natural
Division of Environmental
Health
Wheatly Shopping Center 2
St Croix VI 00802
(809) 777-4577
Fax: (809) 774-5416

VERMONT
VT Dept of Health Asbestos &
Lead Program
108 Cherry St PO Box 70
Burlington VT 05402
(802) 863-7205
Fax: (802) 863-7483

WASHINGTON
WA Dept of Health
Office of Toxic Substances
PO Box 47825
Olympia WA 98504-7825
(360) 753-4035
Fax: (360) 586-5529

WISCONSIN
Bureau of Public Health
1414 E Washington Ave
Rm 96
Madison WI 53703
(608) 266-1253
Fax: (608) 267-4853

WEST VIRGINIA
West Virginia Environmental
815 Quarrier St Ste 418
Charleston WV 25301
(304) 558-2981 x30
Fax: (304) 558-1289

WYOMING
Dept of Health
Preventive Medicine Division
Hathaway Bldg 4th Fl
Cheyenne WY 82002
(307) 777-6951
Fax: (307) 777-5402

Footnotes

(1) All HEPA (high efficiency particulate air) vacuums, by definition, filter out about the same particle size. The HEPA vacs suitable for residential work range in price from about $300 to $1,500. Many of the less expensive models are of high quality and are perfectly adequate. **F** Sufficient study has not been done, but it appears a regular vacuum with a high efficiency filter combined with a lead-specific cleaner **F** works well. Any vacuum you purchase should have a paper throw-away dust bag. It shoud be changed frequently. Read the instructions! Change the filter on a drop cloth. Wear a NIOSH-approved dust mask and cleanup the area after carefully replacing the filter bag.

For residential clean-up work a regular vacuum cleaner can be used but it will work better if a fine particle bag is used. These bags are sometimes called micron or allergen bags.(from pgs. 4, 57, 64)

(2) The Title X Task Force was convened by the Department of Housing and Urban Development in 1995 to develop recommendations for lead-based paint hazard reduction and financing. (from pgs. 20, 73)

(3) There are several good reasons to get rid of wall-to-wall carpets.
• Wall-to-wall carpets can collect large quantities of lead dust and can never be completely cleaned. Area rugs can be sent out to be cleaned and the floor under the rug can be cleaned. If you are going to have wall-to-wall carpets in place, cleaned, professionals with truck-mounted machines do the best work.
• Wall-to-wall carpets hold moisture, which can result in damage to paint and flooring. Area rugs should be hung up and aired out.
• Wall-to-wall carpets collect food particles which attract roaches (a major cause of respiratory disease).
• Having wall-to-wall carpets or rugs in kitchens and bathrooms is extremely unsanitary! Always replace them with cleanable surfaces like vinyl flooring or tile.
• There can be substantial build-up of mold, mildew and dust mites leading to respiratory diseases. Area rugs can be hung out to dry and be sent out for cleaning. (from pgs. 21, 23, 29, 65)

(4) A payment schedule is an agreement to pay the contractor when particular stages of a job are completed to the customer's satisfaction. The larger the job, the more draws of payment. On small jobs, the most a contractor is allowed to request up front is 30%. Hold out something (10% on a small job) until dust tests return below clearance level. (from p. 36)

(5) Air monitoring on large jobs, particularly jobs with potentially hazardous conditions, should be done by an industrial hygienist or other "competent persons" as defined by OSHA. Small residential jobs rarely need air monitoring. The process consists of taking air samples of a particular crew doing specific work measured over an eight-hour day. The samples are sent to the lab, which analyzes the amount of lead in the air. Based on these results, the level of worker protection necessary is determined. The lead level at which respirators must be worn is 50 micrograms per cubic meter ($\mu g/m^3$). A goal may be to keep levels below 10 $\mu g/m^3$ for a particular operation. This exposure is so low as to not need monitoring. Nevertheless, it may be prudent to wear a NIOSH-approved (it says this on the package) if any dust is being created. (from p. 39)

6) A protocol is a description of how to do something. HUD has a protocol for dust testing. **E** It is more stringent and therefore more accurate than the methods described in this document. It includes testing an unused wipe right out of the container (as a base line), changing gloves for every wipe, sending samples in special laboratory tubes, etc. If the dust testing is done for legal clearance, HUD guidelines should be followed. The method outlined in this document is designed to find levels that are lead poisoning hazards. (from pgs. 52, 60)

7) The reason to use a squeezer bucket rather than a wringer bucket is that in a wringer bucket, the mop head is placed between the wringers into dirty water each time it is used. The squeezer bucket holds the the mop head in a basket above the dirty water. (from p. 64)

8) TSP (tri sodium phosphate) cleaners are often recommended but they have three disadvantages:
   • They can burn a person's skin and damage furniture finishes. If mixed too strong they can damage paint.
   • If not completely rinsed they will leave a film that can cause paint failure.
   • They are bad for the environment. They have been banned in some states. You can use strong household cleaners, but lead-specific cleaners **E** work best. (from p. 64)

9) Sanders with attached HEPA vacs may be safe if designed and used correctly. It is recommended that you ask for a small area to be sanded as a sample to see if the machine damages the surface. The operator must wear a respirator at all times. If the machine is used indoors, a dust test taken from under the sample work area, before and after, will provide helpful information. For large indoor jobs, professional air monitoring during a day of work would be useful. See footnote five. (from pg. 43)

Notes

Author & Illustrator

Dennis Livingston is the director and founder of Community Resources, which designs and implements projects that focus on solving urban environmental problems. The foundation for these solutions is creating community controlled, economically sustainable programs. Livingston's work in the field of lead poisoning prevention has included serving on the EPA's Title X Lead-Based Paint Hazard Reduction and Financing Task Force. He was an author and illustrator of the EPA Lead Worker and Risk Assessor Curricula and the National Institute of Building Sciences' Guide Specifications for Reducing Lead-Based Paint Hazards. He serves as an instructor at the University of Maryland Environmental Health Center and has developed dozens of lead prevention and weatherization training programs for municipal employees, neighborhood organizations, property owners and small contractors. As a union carpenter (Local 101) since 1972, Livingston applies his hands-on knowledge of contracting and building skills to his teaching and writing.

Livingston is also a chart designer. He is the originator of the Social Stratification chart (The New Press, NY, NY). He was co-director of a community theater and partner in a cabinet making company. He received his MFA from Ohio University in 1966.

PROFILE OF COMMUNITY RESOURCES. FOUNDED BY DENNIS LIVINGSTON, COMMUNITY RESOURCES WORKS WITH NEIGHBORHOODS TO REBUILD A SUSTAINABLE, COMMUNITY-CONTROLLED ECONOMY IN A HEALTHY ENVIRONMENT. Community Resources provides ongoing consulting, training, materials and program development for neighborhood organizations, small property owners, contractors and municipal and non-profit health, housing and environmental staff.

PROGRAMS INCLUDE:

ADVOCACY AND JOB TRAINING for community organizations.
- Outreach, clean and stabilize training to create healthy and lead-safe homes.
- Organizer training in Section 3 and Environmental Justice compliance.
- Grant writing assistance
- Creating technical training programs for low-income community members to develop technicians, supervisors and skilled trades people.

INFORMATION AND ADVICE for small property owners.
- Training for owners, managers and workers on how to inexpensively integrate lead-safe and other environmental measures into regular turnover and maintenance work.
- Proactive workshops in environmental record-keeping and creating safe work habits that lower costs and frequently make relocation of tenants unnecessary.

WORKSHOPS AND PROJECTS for contractors.
- Marketing environmental remediation as part of home-improvement services.
- Creating job opportunities for contractors from low-income communities including how to negotiate for HUD Section 3 work.
- How-to-workshop on developing a "shared resource" program including overhead, administration, capital equipment, facilities and negotiations with municipal agencies.

SUPPORT AND EDUCATION for municipal and non-profit health, housing and environmental staff and consultants.
- Traning trainers and curriculum development.
- Briefing papers and grant proposals for community-based delivery systems.
- On-site seminars for staff including whole house environmental remediation and implementing cooperative programs with contractors, advocates and property owners.

PUBLICATIONS AND DOCUMENTS including technical illustrations, writing, charts, layout and design. Three recent examples:
- Protocol for a healthy house analysis and remediation program *(Alameda County Lead Poisoning Prevention)*
- A manual for deconstructing and reusing building components *(Institute for Local Self-Reliance)*
- Workbook on Lead Paint in Historic Restoration. *(Illinois Historic Preservation Agency).*

COMMUNITY RESOURCES OFFICE IS LOCATED AT 28 E. OSTEND STREET

BALTIMORE, MARYLAND 21230

E-Mail dlresource@aol.com

Voice (410) 727-7837

Fax (410) 727-4242

For additional copies of **MAINTAINING A LEAD SAFE HOME** *write:*
Community Resources, 28 E. Ostend St., Baltimore, MD 21230

❏ Please send me copies of **MAINTAINING A LEAD SAFE HOME** for $14.00 per copy plus a $4.00 shipping charge for the first book and $2 for each additional book.

Name_____

Organization_____

Address_____

city_____State_____Zip_____

Qty: **Total**   **For Fastest Service,**

_____ **Maintaining A Lead Safe Home $14.00** $_____   **Call (800) 848-0418 or**
      Shipping: $4.00 for first book   **Fax (410) 727-4242**
              $2.00 for each addt'l   _____   *Substantial quantity*
            TOTAL ENCLOSED $_____   *discounts for*
                                                                                          bulk orders
Checks payable to Community Resources

---✂---

For additional copies of **MAINTAINING A LEAD SAFE HOME** *write:*
Community Resources, 28 E. Ostend St., Baltimore, MD 21230

❏ Please send me copies of **MAINTAINING A LEAD SAFE HOME** for $14.00 per copy plus a $4.00 shipping charge for the first book and $2 for each additional book.

Name_____

Organization_____

Address_____

city_____State_____Zip_____

Qty: **Total**   **For Fastest Service,**

_____ **Maintaining A Lead Safe Home $14.00** $_____   **Call (800) 848-0418 or**
      Shipping: $4.00 for first book   **Fax (410) 727-4242**
              $2.00 for each addt'l   _____   *Substantial quantity*
            TOTAL ENCLOSED $_____   *discounts for*
                                                                                          bulk orders
Checks payable to Community Resources

---✂---

For additional copies of **MAINTAINING A LEAD SAFE HOME** *write:*
Community Resources, 28 E. Ostend St., Baltimore, MD 21230

❏ Please send me copies of **MAINTAINING A LEAD SAFE HOME** for $14.00 per copy plus a $4.00 shipping charge for the first book and $2 for each additional book.

Name_____

Organization_____

Address_____

city_____State_____Zip_____

Qty: **Total**   **For Fastest Service,**

_____ **Maintaining A Lead Safe Home $14.00** $_____   **Call (800) 848-0418 or**
      Shipping: $4.00 for first book   **Fax (410) 727-4242**
              $2.00 for each addt'l   _____   *Substantial quantity*
            TOTAL ENCLOSED $_____   *discounts for*
                                                                                          bulk orders
Checks payable to Community Resources